Thriving
WHILE
Disabled

Recognizing Bias

ALISON HAYES

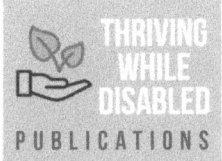

Thriving While Disabled: Recognizing Bias
Author: Alison Hayes

Published by Thriving While Disabled Publications, New Jersey, USA

thrivingwhiledisabled.com

Contact publisher for bulk orders and permission requests.

Copyright © 2025 Alison Hayes

All rights reserved. No part of this publication may be reproduced, distributed, or transmitted in any form or by any means, including photocopying, recording, or other electronic or mechanical methods, without the prior written permission of the publisher, except in the case of brief quotations embodied in critical reviews and certain other noncommercial uses permitted by copyright law.

ISBN (Hardcover): 979-8-9918395-5-6
ISBN (Paperback): 979-8-9918395-6-3
ISBN (eBook): 979-8-9918395-7-0

Dedication

To my mother,

who always taught me to speak up for myself, defended me when I couldn't, and taught me to honor and respect those with different identities and experiences from myself.

Thank you for modeling the work of helping people through laws and advocacy, and helping me understand how good intentions don't always lead to good laws.

I'm forever grateful for your love, trust, and support as I have made my way through life.

CONTENTS

Dedication 5

Quick Note On Using This Book 9

Foreword 17

SECTION 1 » Putting Things Into Perspective 21

CHAPTER 1 » Who is Alison Hayes and where am I coming from? .. 23

CHAPTER 2 » History of the Disabled Identity 29

CHAPTER 3 » Recognizing Ableism 43

CHAPTER 4 » Costs of Being Disabled: Lessons in Classism 57

CHAPTER 5 » Reframing Classism 71

CHAPTER 6 » Social Realities of Disability 81

CHAPTER 7 » Minority Stress: Disability counts too! 103

CHAPTER 8 » Pacing 111

CHAPTER 9 » Disability Culture and Tropes 113

CHAPTER 10 » Practicing Mindful Self-Compassion 135

SECTION 2 » Disability Life Milestones ... 143

CHAPTER 11 » Our Right as a Minority to Exist:
Disabled lives are too often viewed as disposable ... 145

CHAPTER 12 » Citizenship, Immigration, and Disability:
No country wants more disabled citizens ... 159

CHAPTER 13 » Education and Disability ... 167

CHAPTER 14 » Marriage: The financial and social realities ... 192

CHAPTER 15 » Children and Disability:
Risks and rewards as a parent with a disability ... 209

SECTION 3 » Creating a Better Future ... 219

CHAPTER 16 » Disability Rights Advocacy:
Creating a better future ... 221

CHAPTER 17 » Enforcing the ADA ... 227

CHAPTER 18 » Reframing Ableism and
Working to be Anti-Ableist ... 229

CHAPTER 19 » Embracing Universal Design ... 233

CHAPTER 20 » Universal Benefits ... 239

CHAPTER 21 » Thriving With Your Disability IS Advocacy:
What can you do right now? ... 245

Closing Letter ... 251
Next Steps With Alison! ... 254
About the Author ... 255
Glossary ... 259

As of January 19, 2025, the programs and protections listed in this book were current and available.

As these resources may change over time, the author is maintaining an updated vault of information and website links on her dedicated webpage:

thrivingwhiledisabled.com/ twdrecognizingbiasresources

Quick Note On Using This Book

Very often, living with a disability means trying to put out many fires at once while carefully managing your energy.

So, please prioritize your needs, and if you need to, jump to the chapter or section you need most in the moment.

I am American and my examples are primarily from the US. However, much of the experiences around disability and ableism are relatively universal. You will find some specifically US laws discussed at times in this book. If you are not American, you can use these as a starting point to compare with your home country's laws, no matter where you live. I believe that most countries will have similarly ableist presumptions built into them, though of course the details will vary.

Please note that I am neither an accountant nor a lawyer. I am giving you information based on my personal experience and what I have read or heard from others with personal or specialized knowledge. The information I am sharing is often generalized or statistical, so be sure to consult with the appropriate professionals for your specific case if you are uncertain. I cannot know the details of your situation, so please be sure to actively protect yourself and use your best judgment

A word on language and word choice in this book

The meaning and social acceptance of words and word choice evolves over time. It has evolved even more quickly with the use of the internet and increased sharing of information. In some areas I'm discussing (identity groups), words that were acceptable often become passe, and words that were inappropriate sometimes are adopted, adapted, or reclaimed. I am a product of my times.

Within the disability community, multiple debates have raged about both terms to use, and other aspects of language choice.

Use of the terms "disabled" and "disability" have sometimes been subject to debate. To my mind, it is the best option to describe our community, and it is a neutral term. To some people, the terms "disabled" and "disability" feel negative, and they look for alternatives. I suspect that the negative feelings around the terms are mainly a response to the ableism in society and has nothing to do with the words themselves.

We often try to avoid using taboo words or descriptions and attribute negative feelings even to the more clinical or appropriate usage of those words. Do terms like "bowel movement", "urination", "sex", "menstruation", or "period" make you squirm a little? Do you have alternative names for any of these actions? It's the same concept. Taboo topics always to some degree make us uncomfortable. I know there are quite a few alternative words here, as these concepts are somewhat taboo in the US. Alternative words to describe disability like "differently abled" or "handi-capable" are simply attempts to soften the term, or distance it from its origin. Using those terms can feel infantilizing to those of us with disabilities. I do not support any of this, so use "disabled" and "disability" throughout the book, other than when referring to specific subsections of the community, in which case I use what, to the best of my knowledge, is the most acceptable term at this time.

While the actual origin of the term "handicapped" isn't insulting (historically a "handicap" is simply an adjustment in rules based on an individual's experience), it has fallen out of favor in the US, and the term "accessible" has more recently been introduced as a replacement. This change follows the biopsychosocial perspective (discussed in Chapter 2) of shifting the blame or responsibility from the individual to society. "Handicapped" parking is specifically set aside for a person with a disability. "Accessible" parking is generally the closest or most convenient location that anyone can use, including people with disabilities—so the spot is reserved only for people who need that close or easier access, because abled people can use the other spots without being too inconvenienced. The expectation is that if you need those spots, you will go through the appropriate process to access them.

I dislike the term "special needs". It seems to be falling out of favor here in the US. Most commonly, the term is used to describe children with disabilities, especially children with learning, intellectual, or developmental disabilities. I most commonly see it used in relation to the Department of Education, especially to describe school-age and pre-school age children. Teachers who primarily work with these children are referred to as Special Education teachers. I have family members who are Special Education teachers. I was labeled a "special education student", which colored how I respond to this terminology. As an adult, I see the label as overly euphemistic, avoiding the term "disability" as if it's taboo or inappropriate.

I have also seen some neurodiverse people consider embracing the term as an acknowledgement of sensory dysfunction and their risk of sensory overload. In this book, I use the terms "special education" and "special needs" when I'm discussing the education system and related considerations because they are the official terminologies used. I would generally not use the term to apply to an individual with a disability unless they actively told me that was their preferred terminology.

Person-first language (people with disabilities) as opposed to identity-first language (disabled people) is still a hot topic, with divides both in terms of how abled people should describe us and how we should describe ourselves. In this book, I alternate between the two as feels appropriate to me in the moment. This is because there are very strong feelings on both sides, and I understand both perspectives.

The short version is that people-first language has been strongly advocated for over the years, as too many individuals fail to recognize our basic humanity—similar to the person-first language "people of color" used for that identity group. Person-first language is especially supported within the developmental disability and intellectual disability communities (frequently shortened to IDD or I/DD community), as these groups are especially likely to be dehumanized, abused, or neglected. On the other end of the scale, many people within neurodivergent communities have strong preferences for being described using identity-first language (for example, an autistic person, rather than a person with autism). The logic behind this is that, especially for members of the neurodivergent community, their condition and identity are inextricably bound together (the "condition" is an essential part of their identity/personality, and "fixing" it would change their essence as a human being). Others with disabilities commonly argue that the choice of using person-first language reinforces the "othering" of people with disabilities. I'm not sure this is the case, but I do recognize these points.

I often describe myself using identity-first when it comes to disability, though if I share my condition/s, I tend to describe myself as having or having a history with that condition—I'm a disabled person who lives with FND (Functional Neurological Disorder), migraines, and a history of depression and anxiety.

If I was writing a formal paper, I might consistently use person-first language (as that has become the terminology accepted as more socially aware), but in a book it felt most appropriate to alternate between forms—I want to make it clear that I recognize the debate and logic behind these different expressions and my decision for this book is to use both as they felt most appropriate to me at the time of writing.

I do not use the term "able-bodied", as many disabilities are non-apparent. Instead, the opposite of "disabled" is "abled". Disabled people are managing a disability, or a difference in mental and/or physical functionality. Abled people fit normative standards for physical and mental capabilities and emotional lability, while people with disabilities do not. This does include the neurodiverse community—while these differences are not a failure of function but part of the range of human expression, they do not fit abled normative expectations and so are disabled by the failure of society to accept/include them.

Along the same lines, I use the term "non-apparent" rather than "invisible" when describing these disabilities, because the reality is, if you know the person with the disability well, or you are familiar with their condition (or similar ones), you may notice "tells" in their behavior or actions that let you know they are symptomatic or managing symptoms. Invisible implies that there is no way of knowing that they are not abled—and that may also be the case!

Quick Note on Using This Book » 13

The reality is that it's easy for people—especially abled people—to miss the subtle clues of the person's struggle. Again, there has been a push from some members of the disability community to update or switch the terms, but this has not yet become the norm. I feel that "non-apparent" is a more apt term, and so I have chosen to use it in this book. This is a recent change for me, so it's possible I may have missed the phrase at some point in editing the book, but it has been my intention to use "non-apparent" in nearly all cases (the exception being if a group or organization directly refers to invisible illnesses, I do not feel it is my place to change/correct that).

With other communities mentioned in the book, I attempt to be accurate and respectful, whether I am part of the community or not. If I make an error in terminology or use words that you or your community finds offensive or inappropriate, I would love to learn what you feel is more appropriate—and to understand my error. It is not my intent to be disrespectful or dismissive of any identity, and I apologize if I do so in error.

In relation to gender and sexual orientation, my instinct is to use "LGBT" or "LGBT+" to describe that community, and while I know that often a fuller expansion of the acronym is used (such as LGBTQIA), please know I mean no offense, and am accepting and intend to be respectful of all identities. I identify as bisexual, and as part of the greater community, I'm simply using the terms I feel most comfortable with. Fun fact: you can usually tell how old an LGBT+ organization is based on what acronym or terms are used in their name (or the name in their URL)! For example, New York City's LGBT Center's URL is actually

gaycenter.org

due to its relative age as a community center. Getting the B and T added to the name was a struggle, and the bisexual flag flew at the Center for the first time around 2019, and I was privileged to be there and watch the flag being raised!

The term "bisexual" itself is now often unfavorably compared to "pansexual". My interpretation of "bisexual" has always been "attracted to one's own gender and other genders", even though the word "bi" does imply the existence of only two genders. When the term was coined (in the late 1970s), this was the common belief, but the definition of the word has evolved to be more inclusive. While "pansexual" automatically covers that difference ("pan" meaning "all"), it is less often acknowledged by society at large, so I have gone with the more recognizable term whose meaning is more intuitive and easily recognized.

I recognize racial differences in points in the book and discuss minority identities and prejudice. Again, I have heard discussion and disagreement about ideal terms for BIPOC identities, especially when broken down by the individual communities. I have chosen to use the terms that feel most appropriate and at times have used the terms "Black", "BIPOC" ("Black, Indigenous and People of Color"), or "People of Color". I have intentionally not used the term "African American" in most cases as I believe that it is falling out of favor—with the exception being when it is 100% the correct term—and because it specifically focuses on people with a familial history of slavery in the US. There are now a percentage of Black people in the US (and most Black people internationally) who do not necessarily have that history, and the data can be difficult to tease apart.

My partner is Hispanic and Latino and I generally use "Hispanic" referring to him and the greater community as that is the identifying term he prefers. The terms are not synonymous; technically Hispanic refers to any group of people associated with Spain and the Spanish language and culture, while Latino specifically refers to people from Latin America (which includes speakers of additional languages, like Portuguese).

When discussing class and income, I mostly use "low-income" or "poor" as descriptors and recognize that the definition of these terms is relative. I sometimes use the term "poverty" to describe experiences. I do not use any of these terms with judgement in mind, but instead with the goal of naming painful situations. "Low-income" feels like a more politically correct term and is what is preferred by US programs related to poverty. I alternate my usage because "poor" and "poverty" are more accessible and "low-income" feels like another way to add a layer of insulation against a taboo concept. Unless specifically stated, the conversation is focused on relative poverty (poor or challenged in relation to others in the country), rather than absolute poverty (lacking shelter or food).

In expanding my book, I've had to discuss geography and global differences in values, wealth, and support. I tend to use the terms "global north" and "global south", as it's terminology I picked up in graduate school conversations and lectures and other discussions of relative poverty globally. I want to be clear here that the "global north" includes Australia and New Zealand as predominantly white, former British colonies that are part of the industrialized (wealthier) world and culturally much more aligned with them. Another set of terms I've picked up that often describe these areas include the divide between industrialized and non-industrialized, and colonizers and colonized lands. I respect the reasoning behind these terms, and as part of the historical global north/industrialized world/colonizer population, I recognize my position of relative privilege and power. Global north struck me as the most neutral and acceptable term to use, and I've striven to be consistent in doing so.

I do speak in generalities when I'm discussing these topics because it's not possible to do research on all country's attitudes and laws. My point in this book is to differentiate between countries that provide some form of social safety net (which generally fits the global north/industrialized nations/colonizers) and those whose safety nets (if they exist at all) are provided through nonprofit organizations or other non-governmental entities.

This book was initially written as a guide by an American for Americans, so my focus (and expertise) is on laws and government programs that provide support as that's how the US system works. I presume that there will be more parallels in coverage in the global north than the global south and everything else flows from there. I have interviewed people in multiple countries to glean additional information and stories and so it is predominantly my own social network that has been used to collect information. Again, this biases me towards the global north and often people with other similarities to myself. I hope you find this book helpful and useful in your journey.

Foreword

I've been focused on supporting fellow disabled Americans through the struggles that come with being or becoming disabled, and have known for a long time that I wanted to put together a book for this purpose.

Over time, I've heard stories from people in other countries about their disability experiences and have noticed the similarities and seeming universality of emotional impacts, fears, and treatment by others.

The 2024 election results have left me very afraid that the programs I discuss in this book may soon either not exist at all or at least become further defunded so their services become even more limited. I want to be clear: every program I discuss here is at risk due to the election results. This is a time of great uncertainty and fear for me and millions of other people with minority identities. This is a bad time to be anything other than a cis, straight, white, abled, Christian man.

Due to these changes, my original purpose and idea has developed into two books, now a series built on the idea of **Thriving While Disabled**. Volume I, **Recognizing Bias**, (which you are reading now) focuses on painting the picture for you of the current disability experience, including life milestones and steps to improve our future. Volume II, **Navigating Disability Finances**, focuses on practical advice to help you work through the many systems and structures to maximize your opportunities to lead your life as you want.

I have worked to give this volume—and Volume 2 in the series—a more international flavor. The core messaging is the same, as I believe that structural ableism is an international issue, and while many countries have socialized medicine, disabled people remain the people who use the medical system the most and are most likely to experience the biases that exist throughout the medical system.

Ableism appears to be deeply entrenched in all social welfare systems and is a major issue in employment globally. I believe the differences are in the severity of the experience and the level of protections your country provides.

At one time, the US was ahead of things when it came to the rights of people with disabilities. The Architectural Barriers Act (1968), Section 504 of the Rehabilitation Act (1973) and the Americans with Disabilities Act (1990) are three examples of forward thinking in the US. However, since then, things have stagnated a bit, and other countries have caught up or surpassed the protections and rights granted to people with disabilities. Other countries have passed laws that are egregiously ableist or that reflect an ableist bias. I am not aware of any country that has actively and consistently worked to dismantle ableist influences or beliefs. Please educate me if I'm wrong!!

While most of my examples will be American, I will add in more of what I know of other countries' laws, attitudes, and behaviors related to disability or particular programs intended to support us (and/or how badly they may fail us).

I will provide links to further details on the American programs (and programs I am aware of in other countries), as while the rules and processes I discuss here were true and accurate at the time of writing, I'm unsure if they will continue to be so. I hoped that I was catastrophizing the impact of this election on the lives of minority identities in the US, but I appear, unfortunately, to have been correct.

I firmly believe that all of us living with disabilities deserve to thrive, and I believe that it is possible to build a thriving and positive quality of life while managing one or more disabilities. One of our biggest challenges as people with disabilities isn't our disabilities themselves, but the ableism in society. Ableism is a relatively universal issue, though the precise nature and degree and expression of that ableism will vary by culture and law. People with more severe disabilities may have an equal struggle between their disabilities and the ableism in society, but their situation would still be better if the ableism was less severe.

As an American, I'm intimately familiar with how I experience ableism in the US, but from many conversations I've had with others who share my diagnosis (Functional Neurological Disorder) or my identity (a person with a disability) in other countries, many of our experiences are similar despite differences in the nature of the support programs we participate in or need to use in our home countries. I hope that you find the information useful, informative, and helpful in your quest for a better quality of life while managing your disability.

There is, unfortunately, a strong correlation between disability and poverty, both in the sense of disability and ableism causing poverty, and poverty increasing the risk of a person becoming disabled. I will discuss why deeper in the book, but I want you to be aware of the challenge.

The balance of energy and time is an important consideration within the disability community since most of us have fewer usable hours in the day and less energy to use on a regular basis. This means that no matter where in the world we live, advocacy is harder, and structural ableism means we have to fight harder for similar rights and struggle more to get the care we need. This means it costs more money, more energy, and more time to get the same results as abled people in virtually all aspects of life. That struggle is often nearly as debilitating as the medical condition or difference in thought processes or appearance that have us labeled as part of the disability community in the first place!

I highly recommend taking the time to glance through the table of contents for this book. Volume I (this book) is the picture of disability experience in the world today. Volume II is your survival guide. It's intended to be a step-by-step walkthrough to help you manage whatever big challenges you are facing, so you can get the help you need when and how you need it with minimal waste of time or energy. They work together to give you the background, understanding, and practical support you need to thrive while disabled.

The first section of this book gives you the background information and vocabulary to help you process your situation, understand the challenges, and minimize how overwhelming the actual asking for help or protecting your rights steps are (very much a mental process). I'm doing my best to point out potential triggers so you can mitigate them in advance.

Section 2 is intended to help you contemplate the major milestones you may be facing (or may have already faced) with the disabled perspective and extra wrinkles that being or becoming disabled may add (or may have added) to those milestones.

The final section, Section 3, discusses ways that we can make the future brighter for ourselves and others with disabilities (view it as almost a recuperative activity). My intention isn't to give you a to-do list, but simply to help you see ways we really could help our fellow disabled folks find thriving easier than it currently is, and direct you to information resources that can help you stay better informed on disability-related information and perspectives.

I hope that my suggestions and information help you prioritize what needs to be done to help you manage your expectations and give you the best chance of success!

SECTION 1

Putting Things Into Perspective

Why is it so painful to acknowledge disability and ask for help?

CHAPTER 1

Who is Alison Hayes and where am I coming from?

Where I'm coming from

Hi, I'm Alison. I created the blog Thriving While Disabled in 2018, after Al, my life partner of over 13 years, shattered his acetabulum (his second life-altering injury in his life and in our relationship). I managed all his medical care throughout the process, and, unlike the first time I managed his care, he was able to recognize and appreciate what I was doing.

The first injury had been a brain injury caused by a car accident, so there's no blame in that statement. He was not capable of fully recognizing what I did at that time.

Let me back up a little. I have a long history of non-apparent disabilities. My first diagnosis came around the age of three when I was diagnosed with a gross motor skill delay (a disability affecting my control over full-body activities). I was given support, leading to me having long-term issues only with fine motor control. This has translated into my having horrible handwriting, odd ways of gripping pens, pencils, and sometimes utensils, and other mild challenges related to doing things with my hands.

In response, I learned to type at the age of six, utilized my school's "resource room" (special education support), and had a few learning and testing accommodations in school. This, of course, marked me as "other" from very early in my life, so I have been identified as disabled since then—though at the time I didn't think about it that way or use that terminology (and neither did my peers).

I have been managing depression since the age of nine. Anxiety and Functional Neurological Disorder (FND) were added to the mix while I was in college, though my FND wasn't diagnosed until a few years later.

More recently, migraines have gone from being a minor background concern to being a more severe issue.

Throughout this series, I will be sharing my own story as well as the story of my life partner Alvaro who I generally refer to simply as "Al."

I have gathered experiences of other disabled folks which I'll share in varying degrees of detail to help illustrate the universality of these challenges. I am an American, so the central examples are primarily American programs and systems, but I do believe that international readers will relate to many of the experiences here, even if their local laws and processes are different. I will discuss some of these differences throughout the book, as I spent time talking with disabled people globally (though primarily in the global north).

It's important to know I am a white, bisexual, disabled, cis-gendered woman, and grew up in a supportive upper-middle-class family. We have a family history of mental health issues, and one of my sisters experienced a Traumatic Brain Injury (TBI) in her teens.

Shortly after my FND diagnosis, my father fell off a ladder and died of the resultant brain injury. The trauma of losing my father severely worsened my FND symptoms and I was forced to recognize that I could not work again (at least temporarily).

I applied for Social Security Disability a few months after his death and was approved about eight months later. Since then, I have worked a variety of part-time positions, pivoted my career goals twice, become a Geographic Information Systems professional, and received a Master's in Organizational Change Management. My original intended field of study was aquatic ecology.

My partner Al grew up in a supportive family. He's Hispanic, cis-gendered, and straight and his family has had to deal with many more financial struggles than mine.

His experiences along with my graduate school education helped me understand the variations in our lived experiences and gave me the vocabulary to properly explain them. I've spent time learning about privilege and bias. This volume will blend my experiences with my educational background to help you really understand not only how to get yourself through many of the standard challenges, but how to process your emotions around them.

I've found it helpful to be able to name and identify underlying causes, and what I'm giving you is the information you need to get to the root of the challenges and solve them. I'll be sharing helpful resources that will be updated with the most up-to-date details and additional support for you on your journey by means of my website:

ThrivingWhileDisabled.com

Don't worry, there will be links provided throughout to make it easy! I want to help you save your spoons! (I'll explain spoons in Chapter 9.)

Al grew up not identifying as disabled, but living with an uncle who does, and who was primarily supported by Supplemental Security Income (SSI). During my time with Al, he has experienced two permanently disabling events: a traumatic brain injury (TBI) that has left him with a permanent moderate headache, and a shattered acetabulum (hip bone, the socket of the ball-and-socket hip joint), which was rebuilt about a week after the injury but has left him with chronic pain in that joint.

It took a year, but we eventually determined that the osteoporosis that led to this break was caused by autoimmune pernicious anemia, a chronic health condition that more commonly impacts older folks.

His break, and my managing of it, was the inspiration for my blog and business, **Thriving While Disabled.** This led directly to my decision to write this book.

Why I'm writing this book

I recognize that finances and financial concerns are some of the big challenges related to disability and ones that people tend to be very opposed to discussing in detail due to taboos surrounding money (especially the lack of it).

There are many cultural taboos around discussing disability in the first place (more on that in Chapter 2), and even more negativity around being poor (unless that's the start of the story and the person becomes financially successful).

I decided to take the bull by the horns and just write about disability and poverty anyway. I know I had a hard time figuring out how to handle my own disability claim and everything that came with it, and I know that I had a variety of privileges that made it easier for me to handle than it is for most people in similar circumstances.

My father was an engineer and loved exploring and understanding how systems worked. He ensured that I was well-educated on basic personal finances, budgeting, and how to file my own taxes. From that base, I slowly built and rebuilt my financial life as a poor college graduate who could not reliably work due to her disability.

My mother (who has since retired) had a career that started in social work and evolved into becoming a lobbyist for nonprofits (most of which were specifically focused on various disabled identities) and eventually leading to her working for the New Jersey Department of Human Services, where she worked as a legislative liaison. Throughout her career, she focused on poor and/or disabled people and looking at how their lives were impacted by proposed legislation.

Almost every US program I talk about in these books is one that I participated in at some point or other. This is my lived experience. The few exceptions are ones that I either looked into participating in, explored after somebody else mentioned it to me, or plan to participate in, in the future. I'm talking about all these programs because I don't think there is an existing resource that covers this information in one place. In fact, it seems like disability-related services and poverty-related services are usually operated by multiple different providers that don't necessarily communicate well with one another, and this issue appears to be an international one.

It feels like most disability-related programs globally are piece-meal supports that we (disabled people) need to cobble together from all the individual pieces we find. The US Government seems to keep creating programs related to disability under all kinds of different departments, which makes it confusing to navigate. However, this separation may protect the programs from the worst of the budget cuts that can cripple them. If a cut is made, it may affect one program but not all of them at once.

This series is a unique information resource that combines my personal experience with these programs with guidance on how to use them while giving perspective on why all these processes are much more emotionally challenging than they initially sound. I'll discuss the tendency for these programs to be underfunded, poorly enforced, and frequently deprioritized by the people responsible for carrying out these responsibilities.

I have had conversations with fellow disabled folks around the world and recognize that while programs and many details about them differ, the emotions around applying for and using such programs remain very similar, and the barriers to participation frequently mirror one another.

It is an act of courage and an act of self-care to apply for these support programs, but the experience is often harrowing due to structural ableism (discussed in Chapter 3).

CHAPTER 2

History of the Disabled Identity

A (very) brief history of disability identity in the US

One of the challenges of the cultural identity of disability (discussed in Chapter 4) is that we so rarely know or are educated on our history. It isn't taught in schoolbooks, isn't usually passed down from parent to child, and rarely is the topic of discussion even among disabled people, since we are so often socially isolated, and have so many challenges to navigate.

I recently read "A History of Disability in the United States", by Kim E. Neilson, and I highly recommend it. I'm going to do my best to very briefly sketch out some key points from it to give you a better understanding of why our welfare systems work (and fail to work) the ways they do.

Prior to colonization, Native American tribes held various perspectives but overall tended to believe that every person had natural skills and deficits. Disabilities as interpreted by modern society did not exist, as a person born with what we would identify as a disability was simply a difference, and the individual with that difference wasn't othered, but accepted and respected for however they helped support their community.

In the 1600s–1800s, most of the colonizing people with what we'd identify as disabilities were not viewed that way. They worked mostly in whatever profession their families practiced and were cared for by their families in whatever ways were needed.

There were, however, funds created for soldiers who were too disabled to work. War has always been the one "honorable" way to become disabled, and soldiers permanently injured in battle were the most likely to be supported by society.

Most technological advancements for disabled people have occurred shortly after a war, at which point people put effort into creating tools for these soldiers that sometimes spread to others with disabilities.

As time passed, people who were generally held to be inferior or less eligible for rights were painted as disabled by society. Women, for example, were often described as unreliable and weak (at least white women in the well-off families that had power), even though poor women did in fact work as hard as men in many cases.

Part of the mythology around slavery was the concept that Black people's brains were underdeveloped, making them incapable of rational decision-making and unable to see the bigger picture and make well-reasoned plans. This same mythology argued that Black people were often physically stronger, less sensitive to pain, and well-suited to physical labor.

People we now would identify as part of the LGBT+ community were generally painted as either mentally deficient, mentally ill (a label that continued into the 1960s and is part of most homophobic beliefs), or simply immoral (painting orientation as a choice and associating it with other socially unacceptable decisions or behaviors).

For each identity, a different story of disability was developed. But all these minority identities were considered to be disabled and therefore undeserving of full participation in society.

With the Industrial Revolution, more and more work that family units had traditionally done instead became work done in factories and on a larger scale. The needs of the community became focused more and more on the industry it supported, and these industries viewed people as more replaceable and individual employees more like cogs in the machine.

This meant it became more important for each employee to fit expectations (such as having two legs, being able to stand for hours at a time, seeing the objects he was working on, etc.), and less care was given about what happened to the people who didn't fit. People were more disposable and replaceable than ever before. Many of these changes led to more people becoming disabled.

The eugenics movement of the late 1800s and early 1900s exacerbated the problem. Ellis Island was full of inspectors actively searching for signs of imperfections that would lead to denial of entry into the US. There was a definite image of what Americans should be (white, cis, straight, attractive, wealthy, and abled) and a concerted effort was made at the borders to keep people who failed to meet those standards from becoming citizens – the further they were from the ideal, the harder it was to get through.

This included people who may have had a history of being financially successful but happened to look unusual. Disability was too frequently given as an excuse for refusing entry to people who were otherwise undesirable (such as members of the LGBT community).

In the meantime, more people were institutionalized than ever before, and "ugly laws" were passed, where it became illegal to be seen in public if you were disfigured or otherwise failed to meet normative expectations.

In all these cases, it wasn't solely about disability, but also about financial class. If your family was wealthy enough, you weren't labeled as disabled (or were kept hidden away somewhere relatively nice).

If you were poor or part of a poor family, it was extremely easy for you to be dehumanized and penalized for being disabled.

Starting in the late 1940s, disabled individuals and their families started organizing to protect the rights of people with disabilities. Many professions with a high rate of disability (like mining) had strikes or other actions taken by primarily abled workers when cuts were made to funds designed for the families of people killed or disabled while working. Parents of children with disabilities who were prevented from getting an education, lobbied their local school districts to educate their children appropriately. Those same families often pushed for their adult children's right to work, or to prevent those children from being institutionalized. Other abled people were assigned work in various mental institutions and were appalled by the conditions and treatment of the inmates, and they publicized those details. As other civil rights movements happened in the 1960s and 1970s, the disability community (primarily people with physical disabilities) participated and pushed for disabled people to fully participate in society and have access to public systems.

My additional takeaways from US Disabled History

People with disabilities were accepted as part of mainstream society into the 1700s, with their acceptance waning as the industrial revolution proceeded. While disabled individuals in wealthy families generally were cared for, poor disabled individuals had a high likelihood of falling into poverty or otherwise being stigmatized.

As medical knowledge has become more organized and scientific, more and more of the disability mythology around other minority identities has been disproven, reducing at least the overt use of these concepts. Sadly, many of these beliefs still inform societal biases. Too many medical students still believe racist concepts like Black people don't feel pain to the same degree as white people or homophobic ideas like same-sex attraction is unnatural or a form of mental illness.

To this day, mental illness in general is still not treated as being as "real" as physical illness, and to this day people with mental health diagnoses are less likely to be listened to about any health concern they bring forward[1].

Many folks prior to the 1970s with non-apparent disabilities were either undiagnosed, passing as abled in self-defense, institutionalized, or simply didn't recognize that they had a disability. As the disabled identity has become less stigmatized, more people with non-apparent disabilities have been able to embrace their identity as part of the disability community.

---

1   Columbia University Mailman School of Public Health. "Too Often, Doctors Stigmatize People Living with Mental Illness." Columbia Public Health, published October 19, 2023. **https://www.publichealth.columbia.edu/news/too-often-doctors-stigmatize-people-living-mental-illness**.

International Disability History

I'm going to start this with an acknowledgement that my knowledge and research on this topic is much shallower than I would like. To be fair, the topic is quite broad, and much more complex and nuanced than any individual is capable of doing full justice to. I want to acknowledge that the available information is strongly biased towards the global north (US, Europe, Canada, Australia, New Zealand, etc.—the "industrialized nations"), and minimal information is easily available on the global south (so-called developing nations, many of whom are in the Southern hemisphere). I have added references for starting points to delve deeper into the history of many other nations and regions, and I encourage you to dig deeper into the history of your region, if you live outside the US.

The early history of people with disabilities is presumed to be one of "otherness" with disabled individuals being minimized or shunned by their society. While this is the history as told by white colonizers, the ongoing research that archeologists and others are doing, suggests that this was not always the case. From early humans showing healed injuries (meaning they were cared for despite not being able to help others survive for a time) to Vikings like Ivar the Boneless[2], if you search you will occasionally find disabled individuals throughout history, especially if you know how to look for them.

Many of the trends I mentioned above, like eugenics, the industrial revolution, and war being the sole honorable way to become disabled (and therefore the primary rationale for financial support and improved adaptive tools), were relatively global in existence and impact.

Stories of disability as an explanation for inferiority of non-whites followed many colonizers and were inflicted upon many native people, as well as being the underlying argument for sexism and other forms of discrimination we face in modern times.

---

2   Mark, Joshua J. "Ivar the Boneless." World History Encyclopedia, last published May 13, 2024. **https://www.worldhistory.org/Ivar_the_Boneless/**

Poverty became globally associated with many disabilities for similar reasons, with many disabled individuals pushed towards or into poverty by societal bias, and with the likelihood of becoming disabled increasing with familial poverty, as subsistence living would often lead to malnourishment and malnutrition, increase the risk of bodily injury, and would generally be more stressful than living with adequate income, safer working environments, and other privileges that wealthier individuals and their families experienced.

In many countries, concepts of welfare and charity were eventually applied to people with disabilities, again, often intertwined deeply with poverty and old age. To this day, most social welfare programs lump people with disabilities in with either the elderly or poor, or both, depending on the particular service or discount offered.

The modern Disability Rights movement may have started in the United States but has become global in nature. Each country has had their own biases, their own disability rights advocates, and their own unique solutions for the problems that accompany disability.

I believe we all deserve to thrive, but that makes it all the more important that we understand both the challenges and protections that exist in our part of the world, so we can use what we have to give ourselves a better set of stepping stones to give us something resembling economic stability, supportive health care, and other useful supports that can help us catch our proverbial breath and shift from attempting to survive to learning how to thrive, despite the stigma we face.

Be aware that there isn't a fully universal definition of disability, and many countries may define disability slightly differently as well as having distinctions between people who identify as having a disability and people who are certified as disabled (usually "too disabled to work/support themselves") by their government.

The United Nations states that "Persons with disabilities include those who have long-term physical, mental, intellectual or sensory impairments which in interaction with various barriers may hinder their full and effective participation in society on an equal basis with others."[3]

---

3   United Nations. "Convention on the Rights of Persons with Disabilities

Their Convention on the Rights of Persons with Disabilities was put forward December 13, 2006, and is unique in being the only document of that sort created largely by the group of people it was designed to protect. It is intended to be a model for global adoption, so that people with disabilities will not face as much systemic bias and will receive equitable treatment globally.

That vision has yet to occur, of course, but this convention received the necessary votes very quickly, and the UN is using this work to continue to push for the rights of people with disabilities. Interesting fact: The United States of America has yet to sign the Convention's document.

It's well worth your time to understand how your country defines disability and what protections you may be eligible for. Legal definitions and protections are discussed later, starting in the next chapter: Recognizing Ableism.

Perspectives on disability (understanding models)

We all have different perspectives on life, but very often you can divide shared perspectives into mental models of a situation. Very simply, these models are specific lenses or perspectives shared within social groups that define how they view particular identities. This is not a definitive list, but simply the models I felt most useful for our conversation.

The **moral model** of disability is often found within deeply religious or poorly educated groups of people and in many media depictions of disability. It underpins many of the subconscious biases people hold around people with disabilities that they can't or won't identify. According to the moral model of disability, an individual's disability reflects directly on their or their family's moral character. This can be negative, with the disability seen as proof of a person's villainy (think about how many movie villains have some form of disability), karmic retribution for poor or immoral behavior (for example, believing that a woman's child is "simpleminded" because she had an affair), or the result of negative thinking.

(CRPD)." United Nations Department of Economic and Social Affairs. 1 Accessed April 10, 2025. **https://social.desa.un.org/issues/disability/crpd/convention-on-the-rights-of-persons-with-disabilities-crpd**.

A positive framing of this model views disability as a sign of strength, faith, or honor. The statement "God never gives you more than you can handle" covers this well. Similarly, disability may be viewed as a positive reminder that you survived a major life challenge, such as an individual who "should have died" in a car accident, but miraculously survived with permanent damage, or a person who had a deadly disease and emerged with a disability as a direct result. Within media, this is often seen when a disabled person performs an amazing, almost superhuman action despite their disability (like a wheelchair user successfully climbing a mountain, something many abled people will never do).

People who haven't thought much about disability may tend to use the **medical model** of disability. From this perspective, people with disabilities are "broken", and a doctor "fixes" them or brings them closer to healthy and "normal". For example, a person who cannot use their legs to walk is given a wheelchair so they can move around. While this makes some sense when being used by doctors (medical goals tend to be cures or adaptations), it is unhelpful in our general society, as it makes having a disability only the problem of the disabled individual, and it assumes that anything outside of normative expectations is "broken" and normative standards are the ideal.

Many disability rights activists countered the medical model with what is now referred to as the **social model** of disability. According to the social model, disability is an aspect, or part, of a person's identity, much like their gender, race/ethnicity, and sexual/relational orientation. The social model argues that disability is a social construct (defined by larger society) and therefore it is society's responsibility to adjust the environment for people with disabilities. Following the social model of disability, a person on the autism spectrum isn't disabled due to their diagnosis, but rather by how society treats them for not meeting normative standards (like eye contact and other social norms). Instead of holding the disabled person responsible for their disability (as the medical model does), the social model argues that it's society's failure to anticipate the needs of all people that is the problem.

It is the social model that pushes for curb cuts, accessible bathrooms, ramps, elevators, captions, and sign language interpreters. Each of these are accessibility tools that society can provide (or fail to provide) to welcome (or push out) disabled members of society.

The **biopsychosocial model** of disability was created even more recently by the World Health Organization and attempts to combine the medical and social models. It recognizes that our society created the category of disability and has moved people in and out of that category over time. Disability isn't just the impairment or difference in mind or body (what is diagnosed within the medical model), it's how our society responds to it.

The Americans with Disability Act (which I discuss in Volume II: **Navigating Disability Finances**) and other laws in place in the US (and complimentary protective laws in other countries) along with concepts like universal design (which is discussed in Chapter 19) reinforce the biopsychosocial model, where it is society's responsibility to be accessible for all people, whether disabled or not. This model demands that actions be taken to include all members of society, regardless of gender, age, or ability (among other things).

Disability regulations are intended to protect people who fall under the biopsychosocial model of disability, so not only people with diagnosed medical conditions, but people who are neurodiverse, or people with physical differences (such as scars, burns, or simply differences in anatomy). We all face bias due to being perceived as disabled, even if some of us aren't disabled according to the medical model.

Neurodiverse people are social outliers due to a difference in how they process information and communicate, but these "conditions" are now seen as part of genetic expression (by a majority of people well-educated about this identity, at least), not something that needs to be corrected. Society's response to the behaviors is what is disabling, rather than their identity. For those of us with physical or mental differences that fit within the medical model, it remains true that a portion of our challenges aren't our conditions themselves, but the response by society to those differences.

When you look at things from the biopsychosocial perspective, the social construct of disability shifts from being an individual's problem to being a societal one that can be corrected with careful thought and planning, especially once you take the necessary steps to treat and manage your condition.

> I hope that this knowledge helps you shift your perspective on your own symptoms towards models more conducive to your long-term mental and emotional health.

KEY POINTS

- **Historical views** on disability have changed, with disability at times being accepted as part of human experience, and other times treated as some form of defect that leaves people less than human.
- **Moral Model of Disability:** The perspective that disability is directly related to a person's morality. Disability happens for a reason.
- **Medical model of disability:** The perspective that disabled people are broken and medical care fixes the problems.
- **Social model of disability:** The perspective that disability is a social construct, with greater society defining what disabilities are, who is disabled, and what can be done to make spaces accessible for people with disabilities.
- **Biopsychosocial model of disability:** The belief that the social construct of disability is the result of both medical definitions of disability and society's normative expectations.

RESOURCES

Disability History in the US

A Disability History of the United States (ReVisioning History), by Kim E. Nielsen, 2012

Crip Camp. Documentary movie: 2020. Directed by Nicole Newnham and James LeBrecht. Netflix.

Heumann, Judith, with Kristen Joiner. **Being Heumann: An Unrepentant Memoir of a Disability Rights Activist.** Boston: Beacon Press, 2020.

National Park Service. "Early Treatment." National Park Service, last updated August 2, 2021, **https://www.nps.gov/articles/disabilityhistoryearlytreatment.htm**.

International Disability History (places to start)

Nielsen, Kim E. "Disability History." In Encyclopedia of Disability Studies, edited by Gary L. Albrecht, 1-5. Singapore: Springer Nature Singapore, 2022. **https://doi.org/10.1007/978-981-16-1278-7_2**.

United Nations. "Convention on the Rights of Persons with Disabilities (CRPD)." United Nations Department of Economic and Social Affairs. 1 Accessed April 10, 2025. **https://social.desa.un.org/issues/disability/crpd/convention-on-the-rights-of-persons-with-disabilities-crpd**.

World Bank. "Rompiendo Barreras: Inclusión de Personas con Discapacidad en América Latina y el Caribe." World Bank, October 18, 2023. **https://www.worldbank.org/en/region/lac/publication/rompiendo-barreras**

Wendell, Susan. "Disability and the Dilemmas of Difference." The Journal of Medicine and Philosophy: A Forum for Bioethics and Philosophy of Medicine 21, no. 6 (1996): 665-85.

Vanyoro, Kudzaiishe. "Traditional beliefs inform attitudes to disability in Africa – why it matters." The Conversation, April 27, 2020. **https://theconversation.com/traditional-beliefs-inform-attitudes-to-disability-in-africa-why-it-matters-138558**

Chappell, Linda. "Disability in South Africa: A country profile." Human Sciences Research Council, 2000. **https://repository.hsrc.ac.za/handle/20.500.11910/6122**.
Independent Living Institute. "The History of the Independent Living Movement." Independent Living Institute. Accessed April 10, 2025. **https://www.independentliving.org/toolsforpower/tools6.html**.

AIF. "The Slow March of Progress: An Overview of the History of Disability Legislation in India." American India Foundation, November 29, 2023. **https://aif.org/the-slow-march-of-progress-an-overview-of-the-history-of-disability-legislation-in-india/**.

Allodi, Mara Westling, and Sven-Erik Dahlgren. "Attitudes towards people with disabilities: a comparison of students in special education and students in mainstream education." Scandinavian Journal of Disability Research 7, no. 2 (2005): 100-116. **https://doi.org/10.1080/15017410500237326**.

Historic England. "Disability History." Historic England, August 16, 2023. **https://historicengland.org.uk/research/inclusive-heritage/disability-history/**.

Bakkalbasioglu, Esra. "Negotiating Access: The Everyday Lives of Disabled People in the Ottoman Empire." Middle Eastern History 8, no. 2 (2024): 147-164. **https://doi.org/10.1177/16118944241290903**.

Models of disability

Indiana University. "Models of Disability." Indiana University Bloomington, last updated January 26, 2024. **https://accessibility.iu.edu/understanding-accessibility/models-of-disability/index.html**.

American Psychological Association. "Models of Disability." American Psychological Association, 2024. **https://www.apa.org/ed/precollege/psychology-teacher-network/introductory-psychology/disability-models**.

Disabled World. "What are the Models of Disability? Medical vs Social Definitions." Disabled World, last updated March 25, 2024. **https://www.disabled-world.com/definitions/disability-models.php**.1

The Nora Project. "Medical, Social, and Biopsychosocial Models of Disability." Accessed July 8, 2024. **https://thenoraproject.ngo/nora-notes-blog/models-of-disability-1**.

RESOURCES WEBPAGE » CHAPTER 2

CHAPTER 3

Recognizing Ableism

Ableism is the belief that disabled people are inferior to abled people, above and beyond the actual limits that their disabilities cause. Recognizing that certain symptoms cause somebody to use a wheelchair is not ableist. Describing them as **confined** to a wheelchair is ableist because it assumes that wheelchair usage is a negative thing. For many wheelchair users, the chair frees them to participate more fully in society.

Structural ableism is most often defined as failing to provide access or accessibility tools to disabled people. Examples of this include having access only through stairs, which excludes wheelchair users, or only providing auditory emergency signals, which excludes people who are deaf or hard of hearing, or having information only available visually, which excludes blind people and others with low vision.

In the US, a variety of laws have been passed to deal with aspects of these challenges, starting with the Architectural Barriers Act (ABA), which was passed in 1968. This law was the first step towards true accessibility, with requirements for all government and government-funded buildings to be wheelchair accessible (so curb cuts for wheelchair access, ramps, elevators, and doors wide enough to accommodate a chair, and many other physical changes or adjustments to the buildings so that the physical structures would not prevent disabled people—especially wheelchair users—from accessing and using these spaces). Some countries have passed similar laws since then, but this is far from a universal action.

The ABA law required that public spaces be accessible, with the ideal being curb cuts on every sidewalk, traffic lights having auditory signals for when it is or isn't safe to cross the street, ramps or other tools to make all public spaces accessible, and so on. Despite the fact that this law was passed almost 60 years ago, there still are many places in the US that are not fully accessible, and more places that believe they are accessible, but have made dubious design decisions that prevent wheelchair users or others with disabilities from accessing the spaces, at least with the same or similar ease as abled people.

My understanding is that even to this day there are many countries that have not even taken or enforced this type of step, or who only enforce these laws if an individual with a disability needs to access the space.

 **DENMARK**

For example, a friend of mine in Denmark shared a story about a political candidate who was a full-time wheelchair user. He was elected around 2019, and after his election, they finally built a ramp and made the other adjustments necessary for him to be able to enter the government building where his office was located. I'm grateful he was able to run and be elected, but it is a bit rough that that's what it took for the building to be made accessible.

Structural Ableism is not just about physical structures

I (and many others) view structural ableism on an even wider scale, defining structural ableism as including all forms of structures in society that make it harder for disabled people to fully participate.

The definition of structural ableism that we will be using, therefore, includes conceptual structures, like societal culture and laws that paint disabled people as less human or less worthy, or that are built on the presumption of failure being a defining aspect of disability.

I view structural ableism as a parallel form of discrimination to structural racism, in that many of the systems we participate in are biased against disabled people, with that bias woven into the very structure of our modern society.

Structural racism in the US includes historical practices like redlining[4], and current practices like funding public schools through property taxes[5] and the differences in policing in response based on the financial class of an area.

Redlining was literally only permitting African Americans to own property in defined low-income areas (which were often marked on maps using red ink). While the practice is currently illegal, Black families still often have more difficulty purchasing property that white peers could purchase with relative ease.[6]

Because property taxes pay for schooling, poor districts cannot provide as good an education as wealthier districts, and minorities are often pushed into poverty through this conflation of racist practices.

The policing differences I mentioned mean that generally richer and whiter neighborhoods have fewer police officers, and their primary goal is to protect, while poorer and more racially diverse neighborhoods have more police officers who focus on dominating the people who may be perceived as not precisely following the laws. Racism is often impacted by selective law enforcement, where the general (white) population is permitted to break or bend certain laws or expectations without consequences, and people of color taking identical actions find those laws suddenly enforced.[7]

---

4   Sanger-Katz, Margot. "How Redlining's Racist Effects Lasted for Decades." The New York Times, August 24, 2017. **https://www.nytimes.com/2017/08/24/upshot/how-redlinings-racist-effects-lasted-for-decades.html**.

5   Kamenetz, Anya. "How School Funding Formulas Preserve Racial Inequality." NPR, July 7, 2020. **https://www.npr.org/sections/live-updates-protests-for-racial-justice/2020/07/07/888469809/how-funding-model-preserves-racial-segregation-in-public-schools**.

6   Kamin, Debra. "Discrimination seeps into every aspect of homebuying for Black Americans." The New York Times, November 29, 2022, **https://www.nytimes.com/2022/11/29/realestate/black-homeowner-mortgage-racism.html**

7   Staples, Brent. "How Jim Crow Segregation Moved North." The New York Times, May 27, 2018. **https://www.nytimes.com/2018/05/27/opinion/jim-crow-north.html**.

Likewise, structural ableism includes things like the Supplemental Security Income (SSI) marriage penalty (For more on marriage penalties, see Chapter 14), current work culture (discussed in depth in Volume II of this series), a generally infantilizing attitude[8] (I discuss this more deeply in the disability culture section in Chapter 9), the history of police brutality against certain members of the disabled community[9], the fact that the disabled identity is rarely tracked, and even most algorithms are primed to deprioritize people with disabilities[10].

Work culture in many organizations values time seen working over work products (what you did). There is the undeniable fact that disabled people have a higher unemployment rate than abled people (US and EU details next section). Disabled people are frequently looked upon as children or potential victims, so too many organizations and individuals "protect" or "guide" disabled people, as opposed to empowering or respecting us. Police are frequently called if there is any kind of public issue, so they are called when mentally ill or developmentally disabled individuals need support, and too often end up killing them, especially those who have additional marginalized identities[11].

It all reflects society's negative perception of disability and the general preference of most members of society to ignore the existence of disabled people. All this even though over one-quarter of all people

---

8   Tartaro, Mark Daan. "The Damage Caused by Infantilizing the Disabled." Psychology Today, August 18, 2022. **https://www.psychologytoday.com/us/blog/what-will-you-do-when-i-m-gone/202208/the-damage-caused-infantilizing-the-disabled**.

9   Cokley, Rebecca, and Mia Ives-Rublee. "Understanding Policing Black Disabled Bodies." Center for American Progress, June 10, 2020. **https://www.americanprogress.org/article/understanding-policing-black-disabled-bodies/**.

10 Knight, Will. "How Algorithmic Bias Could Discriminate Against People With Disabilities." Slate, February 20, 2020. **https://slate.com/technology/2020/02/algorithmic-bias-people-with-disabilities.html**

11 Lily Robin and Evelyn F. McCoy, "Policing Is Killing Black Disabled People. Centering Intersectionality Is Critical to Reducing Harm," Urban Institute, October 17, 2023, **https://www.urban.org/urban-wire/policing-killing-black-disabled-people-centering-intersectionality-critical-reducing-harm**.

in the US have some form of disability[12], making us the largest minority identity in the country. Globally, the World Health Organization has identified about 15% of the world population as disabled[13], but their definition of disabled is likely much more medicalized and limited. Europe reports a similar occurrence of disability[14] in their general population as in the US, reinforcing my belief.

In the US, disability is stigmatized, but there are more protections than many other countries provide, so many people with non-apparent disabilities have been able to successfully apply for and receive benefits and talk openly about their disability experiences. A good percentage of the neurodiverse community has been able to get diagnosed and learn coping or management skills to help them mask or manage their diversity in expression, and they too have felt empowered to publicly identify as part of the disability community. I know that both diagnosis and symptom management isn't universally available, even in countries that provide universal healthcare.

We are facing an uphill battle for all forms of recognition, and many of society's rules and expectations push us toward poverty. Being poor is too often framed as a personal failure and a signal for society to devalue us even further.

Structural ableism is deeply ingrained in most societies and rarely recognized, mentioned, or discussed. I want you to hold that in your mind while you read this series because it is such an important part of why every aspect of living with a disability is so very difficult.

---

12 Centers for Disease Control and Prevention. "Disability Impacts All of Us." Centers for Disease Control and Prevention, last reviewed August 2, 2023. **https://www.cdc.gov/ncbddd/disabilityandhealth/infographic-disability-impacts-all.html**.
13 World Health Organization. World report on disability. Geneva: World Health Organization, 2011. **https://www.who.int/teams/noncommunicable-diseases/sensory-functions-disability-and-rehabilitation/world-report-on-disability**.
14 Council of the European Union. "Disability in the EU: facts and figures." Council of the European Union. Accessed April 10, 2025. **https://www.consilium.europa.eu/en/infographics/disability-eu-facts-figures/**.

Recognizing the shame and stigma associated with being disabled

There is no shame in being disabled. There is no shame in being poor. There is no shame in getting support from your own government.

And yet I'm sure you winced a little, internally, at one or more of these statements. Disability and poverty both face a great deal of stigma within and outside the United States. Most of the world practices capitalism to some degree, and one of the values embedded in capitalism is value placed upon the ability to earn money, especially on earning more money than the average person. Most employers are biased against employing people with disabilities, especially when they have abled alternatives to hire. Many disabled people struggle to work full time due to structural ableism and the impacts their disabilities have on their day-to-day lives. This is further complicated by medical care primarily being provided during standard working hours, which frequently leaves disabled employees needing to take time off work to receive the medical care required for them to manage their condition/s.

A side effect of the industrial revolution has been an increasing value placed on conformity and normativity, as mass production is easier when the goal is conformity, both in the production process and in the products themselves. While most minority identities don't, by definition, "conform" (more on minority identities shortly), people with physical, apparent disabilities are the largest, most obvious outliers as they often don't fit even some of the defining characteristics of normative human standards, like the ability to see, hear, or walk unsupported. While this does not actually make any person with a disability less human, it does make it easier to recognize just how othering it can be to live with a disability. For some people with non-apparent disabilities, social interactions and expectations can be similarly othering and alien, even if the challenges are less obvious or the otherness less apparent to the outside observer.

Lack of income and nonconformity, both physical and social, have at times been used to dehumanize us or to leave those of us who are poor and/or disabled open to pity or victimhood, rather than to recognize us for what we are: people struggling with an additional—sometimes burdensome—label.

Ableism in Society

We live in an ableist society. We struggle for inclusion on so many levels, from fighting for basic access to buildings, public transportation, and society in general, to fighting stigma, pity, or toxic positivity (we explore this further in the disability culture section of Chapter 9).

Each type of condition has its own challenges, both internal and external, but all of us with disabling conditions (or who otherwise don't fit normative standards) have some aspect of our identities objectified in a negative way or have experienced having our needs ignored or ridiculed.

These issues become even more apparent when looking at employment rates of people with disabilities[15], and how people with disabilities have historically been treated. Many of us have been devalued, institutionalized, or shamed simply for being who we are.

On top of the stresses that our conditions themselves may create, we carry the burden of societal assumptions and expectations—the presumption that our lives are of lower value, our ability to contribute minimal or non-existent, and that our needs far outweigh what we have to offer.

There are few times in recent history when this has been more obvious than with the handling of the Covid-19 pandemic.

People with pre-existing conditions (AKA people with disabilities) were exposed to Covid-19 more frequently (due to exposure to hospitals, medical centers, long-term care facilities, and other places where Covid-19 was treated, people who treated the condition worked, and/or people lived in communal settings), or went without necessary treatments (to avoid interacting with medical staff and resources or because a treatment was considered optional and unnecessary during the worst of the pandemic).

---

15 U.S. Bureau of Labor Statistics. "Persons with a Disability: Labor Force Characteristics — 2024." U.S. Bureau of Labor Statistics, Feb 25. 2025 https://www.bls.gov/news.release/disabl.nr0.htm.

Doctors frequently made decisions about who was or was not eligible for life-saving treatment once infected by Covid-19 through ableist assumptions (such as presuming that having a disability meant one had a lower quality of life) or chose to prioritize (sometimes on a theoretical basis) abled lives over the lives of current patients with disabilities[16]. Covid-19 itself appears to be a mass disabling event[17]. More recently, moves that greatly benefitted the disability community (like the move to remote work by employers in response to the pandemic) are now being put aside in favor of a "return to normalcy" even though the threat of Covid-19 has not actually ended[18] and remote work has proved to be beneficial for many employees, including in terms of productivity[19].

What is Internalized Ableism?

Because society is full of ableist messaging, it's very easy to absorb and believe it. Internalized ableism occurs when a disabled person turns ableist beliefs inward on themselves. This is a frequent occurrence, and something those of us managing disabilities need to be aware of and on the lookout for.

---

16   Lodhi, Taha. "Careless Healthcare: Ableism During COVID-19." HHIVE Lab - UNC Department of English and Comparative Literature, May 18, 2020. https://hhive.unc.edu/2020/05/careless-healthcare-ableism-during-covid-19-by-taha-lodhi/
17   Roberts, Lily, and Rose Khattar. "COVID-19 Likely Resulted in 1.2 Million More Disabled People by the End of 2021: Workplaces and Policy Will Need to Adapt." Center for American Progress, July 26, 2022. https://www.americanprogress.org/article/covid-19-likely-resulted-in-1-2-million-more-disabled-people-by-the-end-of-2021-workplaces-and-policy-will-need-to-adapt/.
18   Roberts, Lily, and Rose Khattar. "COVID-19 Likely Resulted in 1.2 Million More Disabled People by the End of 2021: Workplaces and Policy Will Need to Adapt." Center for American Progress, July 26, 2022. https://www.americanprogress.org/article/covid-19-likely-resulted-in-1-2-million-more-disabled-people-by-the-end-of-2021-workplaces-and-policy-will-need-to-adapt/.
19   U.S. Bureau of Labor Statistics. "Remote work and productivity." Beyond the Numbers, September 2023. https://www.bls.gov/opub/btn/volume-13/remote-work-productivity.htm.

While disabilities create very real limitations, society imposes even more limitations and beliefs about limitations on those of us with disabilities. There are many things that a person with a disability could do if appropriate accommodations are made. However, society tends to be opposed to asking for accommodations for disabilities, even though people constantly are providing other types of accommodations all the time. For example, blind people often don't need the accommodation of lighting in a room, but sighted people are generally provided with the accommodation of lit spaces to live and work in[20]. (Thank you, Haben Girma for that perspective). Too often, society views symptoms of disabilities as embarrassing signs of weakness, which adds shame to the actual challenge that may exist. Asking for help is often framed as shameful because there's this lingering feeling of owing something to, or being in debt to, whoever you ask for help.

Knowing how my FND-related movement symptoms work, I sometimes elect to stay home instead of going to an event because the cost of going would be too high (risk of injury or just too fatiguing), but that doesn't mean that I can never go, just that I need to evaluate my limits each time I go out. I have noticed that even friends who are aware of my condition, will sometimes be overly concerned if I get symptomatic, in part because of the potential for embarrassment that my symptoms (the movements can be very obviously not in the range of "normal" movements) can cause.

For a person who needs a motorized wheelchair, their limits include needing ramps or elevators that can carry that weight and may involve the need of a charging station after however many miles of travel. But it doesn't define their intellectual limits or hand-eye coordination.

Visible conditions can give some clue about the impairments a person has, but there's a huge (and growing) population with recognized non-apparent impairments, which need to be recognized and respected as well.

---

20 Girma, Haben. "We All Need Accommodations (Excerpt from the White House Disability Pride Month Convening)." Haben Girma, August 15, 2024. https://habengirma.com/2024/08/15/we-all-need-accommodations-excerpt-from-the-white-house-disability-pride-month-convening/.

When dealing with anxiety issues, I do my best to recognize when I'm at a high anxiety level and manage it, as well as being extra aware of potential triggers—either avoiding them or anticipating how to minimize the damage—giving myself some extra processing time.

For many neurodiverse people, that acceptance and understanding of difference can be especially important.

The better you can define and recognize your own limitations, the easier it is to ask for the support that you need, instead of having to struggle to make your needs understood. Defining those needs well lets you better recognize when those needs aren't being met so that you can take steps to correct the problem before it becomes insurmountable.

All too often, this whole process doesn't happen, and instead, a person becomes self-critical, blaming themselves for every aspect of the challenges they are facing and viewing it all as their own individual failure. That doesn't help anyone.

By taking the time to recognize what challenges are solely related to your disabling condition, and which are society's response to your disabled identity, you can reduce or remove the feelings of guilt or shame that may prevent you from living your best life, and finding solutions, both internally and externally, to the challenges society throws your way.

KEY POINTS

- **Disability and Work:** Most disability-related programs in US history have required proof of inability to earn as a condition for eligibility, reinforcing the association between disability and economic dependence.

- **We live in an Ableist World:** Our society inherently favors abled individuals, creating many barriers for those with disabilities.

- **Structural Ableism:** Ableism is deeply embedded in our thought processes and institutions, influencing how society views and treats disabled individuals, as well as in physical design of buildings, objects, public transit, and public spaces.

- **Intersection with other Biases:** Sexism, racism, and other forms of discrimination often have ableist roots, further compounding the challenges faced by disabled individuals. Too often, other minority identities focus on their ability, further stigmatizing the disability identity.

RESOURCES

Ableism

Thriving While Disabled. "Accessibility is About More than just Ramps and Captions" blog post, webpage https://thrivingwhiledisabled.com/accessibility-is-about-more-than-just-ramps-and-captions/

Thriving While Disabled. "Self-Evaluation, an alternative to New Year's Resolution" blog post, webpage: https://thrivingwhiledisabled.com/self-evaluation/

Disabled World. "Neurodiversity." Last modified February 15, 2023: https://www.disabled-world.com/disability/awareness/neurodiversity/.

National Center for Biotechnology Information. "Structural Ableism: Understanding and Addressing Disability Discrimination." Accessed July 8, 2024: https://www.ncbi.nlm.nih.gov/pmc/articles/PMC10770745/.

Healthline. "What is Ableism? Understanding Disability Discrimination." Accessed July 8, 2024: https://www.healthline.com/health/what-is-ableism.

American Psychological Association. "Medical Bias Against Mental Illness." Accessed July 8, 2024: https://psycnet.apa.org/record/2008-11097-001.

Thriving While Disabled. "Recognizing and Countering Ableism from Friends or Family." Accessed July 8, 2024:: https://thrivingwhiledisabled.com/recognizing-and-countering-ablism-from-friends-or-family/.

Thriving While Disabled. "Disabled People Can Practice Ableism Too." Accessed July 8, 2024. https://thrivingwhiledisabled.com/disabled-people-can-practice-ablism-too/.

Thriving While Disabled. "Ableism in Society: Everybody Wants You to Be Okay." Accessed July 8, 2024:: https://thrivingwhiledisabled.com/ableism-in-society-everybody-wants-you-to-be-okay/.

Positive Psychology. "Self-Efficacy." Accessed July 8, 2024: https://positivepsychology.com/self-efficacy/.

Systemic Racism

"Black Disabled Lives Matter." Thriving While Disabled, May 26, 2020. https://thrivingwhiledisabled.com/black-disabled-lives-matter/.

Human Rights Careers. "16 Examples of Systemic Racism." Human Rights Careers, last updated January 29, 2024. https://www.humanrightscareers.com/issues/examples-of-systemic-racism/.

Quillian, Lincoln, Devah Pager, Ole Hexel, and Arnfinn H. Midtbøen. "Hiring Discrimination Against Black Americans Hasn't Declined in 25 Years." Harvard Business Review, October 11, 2017. https://hbr.org/2017/10/hiring-discrimination-against-black-americans-hasnt-declined-in-25-years.1

Annals of Emergency Medicine. "Racial Bias in Emergency Departments." Last modified August 2009. https://www.annemergmed.com/article/S0196-0644 (09)00243-1/fulltext.

Disability and Law Enforcement

Ruderman Family Foundation. "Media Coverage of Law Enforcement Use of Force and Disability." Accessed July 8, 2024: https://rudermanfoundation.org/white_papers/media-coverage-of-law-enforcement-use-of-force-and-disability/.

Police Brutality Center. Accessed July 8, 2024: https://policebrutalitycenter.org/.

Algorithms and bias

SpringerLink. "Moral Agency, Epistemic Agency, and Epistemic Institutional Injustice: Defining and Contextualizing Algorithmic Bias." AI & Society 37 (2022): 667-680: https://link.springer.com/article/10.1007/s10676-022-09633-2.

The White House. "Algorithmic Discrimination Protections." Last modified October 4, 2022: https://www.whitehouse.gov/ostp/ai-bill-of-rights/algorithmic-discrimination-protections-2/.

Journal of International and Comparative Law. "The Impact of Algorithmic Bias on the Administration of Justice." November 2021: https://www.jicl.org.uk/storage/journals/November2021/ShnKBm87YxQCmZpggSqz.pdf.

Covid-19 and employment

Agrawal, Pooja K., Michelle L. Bishop, Adriane Casalotti, and Brian C. Castrucci. "The Impact of COVID-19 on People With Disabilities: Evidence of Disproportionate Health Outcomes." Disability and Health Journal 15, no. 2 (2022): 101247. **https://doi.org/10.1016/j.dhjo.2022.101247**.

U.S. Bureau of Labor Statistics. "Remote work and productivity." Beyond the Numbers, September 2023. **https://www.bls.gov/opub/btn/volume-13/remote-work-productivity.htm**.

Slab. "Does Remote Work Increase or Decrease Productivity?" Slab, February 22, 2023. **https://slab.com/blog/remote-work-productivity/**.

Forbes Technology Council. "The Impact Of Remote Work On Productivity And Creativity." Forbes, January 14, 2022. **https://www.forbes.com/councils/forbestechcouncil/2022/01/14/the-impact-of-remote-work-on-productivity-and-creativity/**.

RESOURCES WEBPAGE » CHAPTER 3

CHAPTER 4

Costs of Being Disabled
Lessons in Classism

REALITY CHECK: It really is more expensive to be disabled

I want you to take a moment to process this: having a disability is physically, financially, and emotionally more expensive than being abled. Let that soak in for a moment.

> 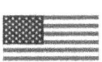 **UNITED STATES OF AMERICA**
>
> While in the US, thoughts immediately jump to financial costs and debt related to healthcare, this is far from the only cost involved. Here in the US, we do bear more of the financial burden related to healthcare than other countries in the global north, and our country's healthcare system is beyond broken. National healthcare plans are generally more affordable and provide better coverage to most people, including people with disabilities. Disabled people in other countries with single-payer healthcare don't have as many healthcare-related expenses as we do in the US.

However, many of these countries have completely different and separate systems for accessibility tools, in-home support, and medications. Some of these are more expensive financially. Others may be emotionally more (or at least similarly) taxing to receive, apply for, or prove eligibility for.

I have yet to have a conversation with anybody who argues that it's less financially expensive to have a disability than to be abled under similar circumstances. Living with a disability is financially more expensive than being abled.

Most people with disabilities end up relatively poor, often below their country's poverty level (I dive into defining poverty in **Navigating Disability Finances**), due to the combination of expenses and lack of income.

Even if those of us with disabilities are able to get full time, permanent employment, we spend more money on our medical care than abled people do (especially here in the US where we need to pay for our health insurance), may need to purchase accessibility tools (some of which are quite expensive), and often have less energy to do things before or after work.

This means that even earning the same income as others, we have less money available for any leisure activities we may want to have. We have less leisure time, as we generally have fewer usable hours in our day, because of the extra time it takes to manage symptoms, daily living taking extra time or energy, or the extra hours of sleep that are necessary for our health.

Our bodies don't really differentiate between physical and emotional stress[21,] so worrying about our finances (or other stressors) can have a negative impact on our health. As people with disabilities, we must handle our financial, mental, and physical health by keeping all our stresses as low as possible. It's very hard to do, but my goal throughout the book is to help you to do so.

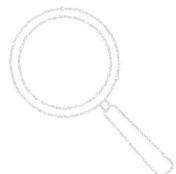

---

21 Cleveland Clinic Medical Professional. "Stress." Cleveland Clinic, last reviewed March 4, 2024. **https://my.clevelandclinic.org/health/articles/11874-stress**.

Recognizing the shame and stigma placed on poverty

Capitalist culture places a huge value on employment and work. Think about conversations you've had—how often has somebody used "What do you do for a living?" as an opening question? The assumptions here are that 1) you are employed and 2) employment is how you provide value to society. While this is particularly true in the US, I believe that discussion around work and employment (which is how most people spend about one-third of their time during their working years) takes up a large portion of many people's thoughts, especially people with more privileged backgrounds.

In this work-focused culture, too often, being poor is viewed as a moral failing, rather than just an unfortunate situation. Too often, it's assumed that if the poor individual just worked harder or tried more, or wasn't so lazy, then they wouldn't be poor any longer. Poverty isn't a moral failing. It's a policy choice. It's something that happens to people due to any variety of challenges in life and is unavoidable when there are so many jobs that don't pay a living wage[22]. Again, the living wage issue is likely worse in the US than it is in many other countries that have a more robust social welfare system or stronger unions (or both), but this underscores my point. Poverty is the result of a government's mismanagement of funds, or the country's lack of funds in the first place.

Intergenerational passing of wealth (inheritance) magnifies many of these issues, with those whose families were wealthier receiving additional benefits (like healthier, more reliable meals, better education, and greater financial stability), while those who weren't born into well-off families are often managing additional traumas (like eviction, food insecurity, and lack of support for struggling family members).

Racist practices have made it even harder for poor Black people to escape poverty in the US. Even the wording I'm using here shows how much negativity being poor has been steeped in. We "escape" poverty as if it's an entity that is actively hunting us.

---

22 Massachusetts Institute of Technology. "Living Wage Calculator." Living Wage Calculator - Massachusetts Institute of Technology. Accessed April 10, 2025. **https://livingwage.mit.edu/**.

The reality is that before Covid-19, 40% of Americans were one missed paycheck away from financial disaster[23]. I suspect that the number of poor people in the US has gone up dramatically since then (or would have, had they survived Covid-19, which disproportionately impacted minority identities, especially folks with disabilities).

The shame and stigma of applying for social welfare support

Applying for needs-based (low-income) programs often takes on a shameful tone, with many viewing poor people as "living off us taxpayers" and other negative connotations.

This is especially true in the US, where the story of picking oneself up by the bootstraps is very popular. While the degree of disdain may vary among countries, I doubt there are many where being poor enough to need government funding to survive is viewed as proof of social success. Most countries in the global North have some form of program to provide disabled people who are unable to earn a substantial income with a stipend to help them survive and have additional programs to help their country's defined low-income population to get by until they can improve their financial situation (I have chapters about these programs in **Navigating Disability Finances**).

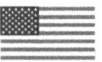 **UNITED STATES OF AMERICA**

In the US, these social welfare programs include TANF (Temporary Assistance for Needy Families), SNAP (Supplemental Nutrition Assistance Program), LIHEAP (Low Income Heat and Electric Assistance Program), Medicaid, and more, with disabled people specifically covered by Social Security Disability Insurance (SSDI) or Supplemental Security Income (SSI) coverage.

---

23 Ivanova, Irina. "40% of Americans are one paycheck away from poverty." CBS News, May 15, 2024. https://www.cbsnews.com/news/40-of-americans-one-step-from-poverty-if-they-miss-a-paycheck/.

If your household's sole or primary source of income is SSDI or SSI, you will, by definition, be low-income (poor) because these programs provide limited payouts.

Many people see even applying for SSDI or SSI as a form of failure. It's an acknowledgment of your own inability to maintain anything resembling a full-time job, which is painful. (Don't worry, I have a much more detailed discussion of this in Volume II of this series.) This is especially true because, due to capitalism, our value to society is primarily determined by our ability to earn money.

Carrying through with the application is basically taking step after step to prove that you aren't capable of working regular hours, convincing those reading the application of your own inadequacy as a human being—with medical notes and statements from your medical care providers to back up your claim—because the concern that you are trying to cheat the system is much higher than any empathy for your challenges.

If you need to see one of Social Security's doctors to be evaluated, the doctor may be focused on disproving your disability (and the limitations that go with it) rather than on how you are doing or how impacted your life is by your condition.

There likely are some doctors who are exceptions to this, but they are not the majority.

These programs seem to work from the assumption of "lying until proven otherwise" rather than the "innocent until proven guilty" that our country states as an ideal.

Most of the government employees responsible for managing these programs are bureaucrats—and those who care quickly become overwhelmed and burned out.

Since these employees are also people, they often carry with them the same association of stigma and/or discomfort with disability and disapproval of poverty that much of the population has. This means the people they are being paid to help often immediately rub them the wrong way simply because they are poor and/or disabled. This doesn't lead to the best possible treatment.

Many people applying for programs/benefits feel humiliated or worthless, and the people processing their claims may reaffirm those feelings, especially when the applicant is another type of minority.

Like most government forms, these applications need to be filled out precisely and the forms are created using certain assumptions, so anything that falls outside of the norms becomes difficult to justify or prove. I share examples of AI and my experience of this and SNAP benefits in Volume II of this series. This isn't an isolated problem. It has occurred for many people in different forms, and it is extremely exhausting.

The social cost of the stigma against social welfare

Many people on social assistance programs don't want others to know. It goes back to that stigma of being poor. If you're poor enough to get SNAP benefits, live in low-income housing, or are living on SSI income, then explaining that is acknowledging your position of relative poverty.

There's a big fear of being rejected by whoever you are talking to. That combination of shame and fear means that many folks on these programs have a hard time openly communicating with new people, and likely a hard time conversing with people who knew them when their financial situation was better.

Inevitably, this other person may ask, "What do you do for a living?" or other painful questions, and the fear of rejection looms large. To move forward in life, people in poverty need to find good work—fear and decreased interaction often cost a person job opportunities, a support network, and impact in other more subtle ways.

Those of us living with disabilities often need to deal with the stigma of being in poverty on top of the stigma of being disabled. This stigma and these fears are hard to get past—and are often reinforced during the process of applying for the very aids we're embarrassed to need.

The thing most damaged in all of this is our **self-efficacy**. Self-efficacy is the belief in our own ability to successfully do things. This belief is frequently viewed as confidence and is generally considered essential for employment.

> **I remember when I first applied for SSDI, I had periods of feeling like a failure.**
>
> Even though I applied after successfully completing a demanding college course load and spending close to a year on a self-financed trip to Australia, I still felt pretty worthless for a while.
>
> I lost several jobs due to my FND symptoms before applying for SSDI, and with those employment losses, followed by my father's sudden death, I knew I wasn't capable of trying again at that moment.
>
> I did everything I could to maintain my self-esteem, but I still fell into a deep depression, and it took a lot of work to get myself back on course.
>
> Once I decided on my career change and started studying, I slowly regained some confidence, but I remember being very shy and quiet at most of the jobs I was able to get.
>
> I was fearful of failure and fearful of making mistakes, afraid that my symptoms would suddenly leave me incapable of completing my responsibilities.
>
> Those fears were debilitating in and of themselves. I know I've lived a relatively privileged life, growing up in a family that could afford to give me many financial and social advantages, as well as having had a college education prior to needing to go on SSDI. I'm aware of these privileges and yet it was still an emotionally challenging process, and those applications were very challenging to complete!

Whatever your situation is, applying for disability-based benefits is going to be a painful and difficult experience, and will shine a light on some of the worst experiences of your life. That doesn't mean it's not worth doing, but I do want you to be prepared, and to understand that much of why it is so hurtful is because of all of the societal messages we've internalized.

Classism in the Law

The US (and likely other countries) has a classist way of creating and reforming laws. If an organization isn't in compliance with a law, the person or people who were damaged by that failure need to prove that the law wasn't followed, generally by suing the organization. This requires documentation and lawyers, both of which require a lot of time, money, and/or energy by the people who sustained the damage.

Once they start this process, the lawyers need to be paid, there are often waits between every step, and of course, the opposing side hires lawyers and provides their own documentation of how they were in compliance, how the failure wasn't their fault, and/or how the person who sued them doesn't have the right to do so. Altogether, this means that a good percentage of the time, whoever has more money has a better chance of winning the case (or at least getting the other side to drop the case or accept money for the damages, which can amount to the same thing).

The process of suing organizations for noncompliance is hard for anyone, but when living with a disability, it is especially difficult because so many individuals and organizations are biased against people with disabilities, including the very organizations supposed to be helping us. When the cultural norm is inaccessibility, it's hard to fight battle after battle for access. Since there is so much bias, and the bias is so severe, the failure needs to be even worse or have an even higher cost to the individual to have a chance of winning.

Because bias against disabled people is so strong, we're even more likely to be poor and have less energy available for things beyond survival.

Like any other minority identity (we'll discuss minority identities in Chapter 7), we have the best chance of success when the damage is severe, when others can sympathize with us, when the immorality of how we are treated is most obvious, and/or it costs people very little to support us. Each of these is extra challenging with disabilities.

We are too frequently dehumanized by society, or painted as children, unable to make our own decisions. Have victories been won? Absolutely—it's not impossible. There's just an extra degree of challenge, and we are behind most other identities in terms of recognized legal rights.

For example, members of the disability community in the US do not have marriage equality due to the way SSI benefits are run. Everyone on SSI is either disabled or over 65 years of age. It simply didn't occur to lawmakers that people eligible for SSI might even want to get married. It didn't occur to lawmakers to adjust asset limits for SSI based on inflation, which is why the asset limits are so woefully low. How low? An individual collecting SSI benefits cannot have more than $2,000 of assets (if adjusted for inflation, the limit for an individual would be closer to $10,000), and a couple is only eligible for SSI benefits if their assets are below $3,000. There currently are proposed laws to correct these issues (discussed in detail in Volume II), but there is very little political will to pass them.

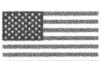

UNITED STATES OF AMERICA

The US disability community only recently won the right to choose how independently we live. The Olmstead Decision[24] in 1999 finally acknowledged that disabled people have the right to choose to live within our community rather than be institutionalized, while still receiving state-funded support. This has been viewed as one of the most important civil rights laws for people with disabilities.

People who create laws and work out their intricacies are usually abled and relatively wealthy. They are used to thinking a certain way and generally do not have the lived experience of the potential negative impacts of these laws. Whether it's failure to consider long-term impacts, incorrect assumptions, or creating a system more concerned with ticking boxes for eligibility than helping the people who need the services, the legal system frequently fails to support disabled people.

---

24 The Olmstead Rights Enforcement Project. "About Olmstead." The Olmstead Rights Enforcement Project. Accessed April 10, 2025. **https://www.olmsteadrights.org/about-olmstead/**.

If you go into the process of getting support knowing these facts, you may be angrier than you would otherwise be, but you'll be much less likely to blame yourself if things go wrong.

I want you to be prepared for these challenges so that every step along the way, you know how little of this is your fault, and you'll be better prepared for the poorly worded questions, the rejection loops, and the slow responses you will face. I want you to remember that while it may be your responsibility to get onto the correct programs or reference the appropriate laws, it is not your fault that it takes up so much of your precious time and energy to do it!

KEY POINTS

- **Classism:** Society tends to view poor people as inherently less worthy, and paint poverty as a moral failing rather than the result of policy decisions by the government.
- **Stigma on social welfare:** Because of classist beliefs, using social welfare programs is generally stigmatized and people on these programs are often shamed for doing so.

RESOURCES

Classism

Desmond, Matthew. **Poverty, by America**. New York: Crown, 2023.

Poor People's Campaign. "The Souls of Poor Folk: A Preliminary Audit." Accessed July 8, 2024: **https://www.poorpeoplescampaign.org/resource/the-souls-of-poor-folk-audit/**.

Poor People's Campaign. "Poor People's Moral Budget." Accessed July 8, 2024: **https://www.poorpeoplescampaign.org/resource/poor-peoples-moral-budget/**.

Poor People's Campaign. "Pandemic Report." Accessed July 8, 2024: **https://www.poorpeoplescampaign.org/pandemic-report/**.

Poor People's Campaign. "Costs of Poverty Fact Sheet." Accessed July 8, 2024: **https://www.poorpeoplescampaign.org/resource/costs-of-poverty-fact-sheet/**.

Shaw, George Bernard. "Poverty as a Moral Myth." The Guardian, October 18, 2017: **https://www.theguardian.com/commentisfree/2017/oct/18/george-bernard-shaw-poverty-moral-myth**.

Eurostat, "Disability statistics - financial situation - Statistics Explained," Eurostat - Statistics Explained, last updated July 2024, **https://ec.europa.eu/eurostat/statistics-explained/index.php?title=Disability_statistics_-_financial_situation**.

Systemic Inequalities

Imogen Calderwood and Erica Sánchez, "There's Finally an Internationally Agreed Upon Definition of Sexism. Here's Why That Matters," Global Citizen, April 1, 2019, **https://www.globalcitizen.org/en/content/sexism-definition-council-of-europe-equality/**.

Center for American Progress. "Systematic Inequality and Economic Opportunity." Accessed July 8, 2024: **https://www.americanprogress.org/article/systematic-inequality-economic-opportunity/**.

Rooted in Rights. "It's Time to Stop Ignoring the Intersections of Marginalized Identities." Accessed July 8, 2024: **https://rootedinrights.org/its-time-to-stop-ignoring-the-intersections-of-marginalized-identities/**.

Scientific American. "How to Think About Implicit Bias." Accessed July 8, 2024: **https://www.scientificamerican.com/article/how-to-think-about-implicit-bias/**.

National Center for Biotechnology Information. "Evidence and Research Needs for Eliminating Explicit and Implicit Bias in Healthcare." Accessed July 8, 2024: **https://www.ncbi.nlm.nih.gov/pmc/articles/PMC9172268/**.

Thriving While Disabled. "Ableism and Racism in Medical Care." Accessed July 8, 2024: **https://thrivingwhiledisabled.com/systemic-racism-and-ableism-in-healthcare/**

RESOURCES WEBPAGE » CHAPTER 4

CHAPTER 5

Reframing Classism

**Reframing the classist perspective:
We all use social welfare programs!**

It's interesting we often have a negative reaction to the name "social welfare" because society has conditioned us to associate it with poverty and being in need, along with all the negative connotations that accompany those circumstances. The reality of the situation is very different from this perception. When you take a step back, it becomes obvious there are many programs designed for the wellbeing of our society that we all benefit from.

Our whole society benefits from the design of public goods like parks and public transportation networks. Schools and other community institutions are designed for social welfare, as living in a community of educated adults helps society function, and that's only done by educating all children, not just the children of wealthy parents. By educating all citizens, we improve everybody's quality of life. People who don't have children or no longer have school-aged children benefit as educated young adults join our workforce able to do the complicated jobs that exist today. Public transit systems help equalize travel opportunities and reduce traffic congestion. Parks add oxygen to the atmosphere and create spaces for our community to gather and enjoy nature, play sports, and allow children (and adults) to run and play.

> 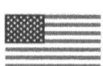 **UNITED STATES OF AMERICA**
>
> Taxes often have loopholes that contribute to social welfare by making exceptions for certain expenses, donations, activities, and decisions. Tax credits are part of the social welfare system, as are mortgage rebates and most other exemptions or credits. The stimulus packages in response to Covid-19 were forms of social welfare.
>
> Federal college loans are social welfare, as are most other government loans. Loans allow adults to attend college and (presumably) use their education to find a career path they love and gain the specialized knowledge to follow that path. Loans help businesses grow and flourish, and organizations expand to better cover those who need them.
>
> The crucial difference between these programs and social welfare support for low-income and disabled people lies in perception. Programs related to taxes, or those recognized as part of an attempt to "better oneself", are socially acceptable, often encouraged. In contrast, needs-based social welfare programs carry a stigma of dependency and failure.
>
> To challenge this classist perspective, we need to recognize that everyone benefits from social welfare programs in some form. Whether it's public education, tax credits, SNAP benefits, or federal loans, these programs (ideally) provide opportunities and support to all members of society.

Why applying for support feels so hard

The low-income programs you may need to apply for are not available through a tax-based model because many of these programs are there to help in emergencies, which generally don't line up with tax season.

If you would normally pay taxes (some of us are too poor to even need to file), you wouldn't want to wait until tax season to get the support you need. Many folks who are eligible for these programs can be so low-income that they don't need to file taxes (I don't need to file unless I earn additional money, as opposed to only collecting my SSDI benefits).

You need to apply for these programs when you recognize that you're in a financial crisis. These are stressful times.

Times of crisis tend to make being organized more challenging, all interactions more stressful, and thought processes and our ability to plan muddled. In other words, you need to apply for social welfare support, by definition, when you are already in a stressful and challenging situation.

To make matters worse, many of these programs are run by different government departments or programs. Each needs-based program has slightly different requirements and often has confusingly worded rules. As these programs only support poor people, they are frequently targeted for budget cuts (thank you, classism).

Due to limited funding and the number of people needing the services, there tend to be relatively long waits during each step and slow response times. If this isn't a setup for disaster, I don't know what is.

Setting your expectations for government supports

Applying for help (don't worry, I give you details about how to apply in Volume II of this series, **Navigating Disability Finances**) can really damage your mental health for all the reasons listed above. You want to be able to approach this realistically and keep a level head when things get stressful. Setting your expectations in advance will help with this.

Just like any other time you participate in a government process (like filing taxes or visiting the Department of Motor Vehicles), expect there to be waits, annoyances, and less-than-polite people.

Understand that these applications won't be emotionally easy, as you are going to be sharing painful information (either details on the impact your disability has on your life or your current financial situation). It's going to hurt to see it all on paper (or on-screen).

If you were doing well, you wouldn't be applying for these programs.

Make sure that you provide everything you possibly can in the form requested whenever you fill out an application.

Even if it takes an extra day or two, providing precisely what is requested increases your chances of having your application accepted the first time, and the processing of your application is often the step that takes the longest.

I have learned that, usually, even when I think I have everything they need, there always seems to be something that they won't accept or that isn't complete enough, so I have to come back, mail, fax, or (if I'm incredibly lucky) email them this one last piece of information.

This is normal.

Again, they tend to be very precise in their requirements and you need to do things the way they insist if at all possible.

Recognize that, in this process, the people who are supposed to be helping you view themselves as gatekeepers and you as a potential liar.

You need to document everything and provide exactly the information they want.

Be aware that while this is very important for you, these people are processing this type of information all day, every day.

Just like in any job, information may get misplaced or lost. In fact, since these folks are government employees and generally in departments that are not well-funded, you can expect that something is likely to go wrong at some point in the process.

If you go in expecting and anticipating this challenge, your surprises are more likely to be pleasant ones.

When applying for benefits, focus on your goals

Focus on the end result. Generally, these programs provide you with money or its equivalent, so focusing on the end goal may help you keep going.

As an example, applying for Supplemental Nutrition Assistance Program (SNAP) lets you better nourish yourself, and Low Income Heat and Energy Assistance Program (LIHEAP) reduces or removes your heating and electric bills, letting you use your money elsewhere.

If you start getting frustrated, remind yourself why you're doing it—so you can eat better, keep the heat going, or live independently. Whatever it is that a specific program will do for you, focus on that outcome as you fight for it. Since these programs will generally cover you for a year or more once you get on them, it's worth the effort to ensure that you get the help you need and deserve.

Above all, realize that, for the moment, using these programs is your job—and you deserve credit for recognizing your own needs and limitations. Once you've got these supports, you can focus on healing yourself and figuring out your next steps in managing or improving your life.

You have every right to these supports (you proved that in your application process) and using them is getting you one step closer to a better life!

Structural ableism and classism are barriers, but you can still succeed!

Over the years, I've taught myself not to be embarrassed.

I've learned to recognize the challenges these systems cause, and I've learned to push back on others' expectations—but it took a lot to get there.

I have always been an outgoing person, an extrovert, and a person who is much more likely to overshare than leave things out.

I now intentionally share that I'm living on SSDI. I intentionally talk about my FND symptoms and how they impact me. I try to talk about difficult subjects like poverty, racism, and ableism because I'm not afraid anymore.

I've met enough people who accept me for who I am that I'm willing and able to take these risks with strangers. I only do so in settings where I feel I am not at risk of an extreme reaction. At times I'm feeling strong enough. In ways that don't put me at risk.

I still find myself preparing for these reveals by talking about what I am doing—I'm running a blog, I'm building a business, and I'm spreading awareness of FND.

I start with that—and the conversation shifts, and we end up discussing discrimination or how broken the social welfare system is or the devaluing of the labor of women.

I share my lived experience of being disabled, of being on SSDI, of applying for SNAP or LIHEAP.

Sometimes people thank me for giving them insight, sometimes people ask me for advice, and sometimes the subject gets dropped.

But it's taken me a long time to get there, and I still am putting a lot of energy into trying not to be viewed as a "drain" on society, rather than simply focusing on my humanity being the thing that makes me worthwhile, worth respecting, and worth protecting.

We all deserve to be treated with respect, and we all deserve to get the support we need. We all should be respected simply due to our humanity.

But we've all absorbed the societal story of poverty as proof of moral failings and disability making us a burden.

We're starting from that assumption too often and fighting for our right to be recognized from the presumption that we aren't a burden.

I celebrate each step forward in this understanding and do my best not to take any steps backward.

You likely have the instinct to feel some degree of shame around being disabled and about being, becoming, or appearing poor. The underlying fear is natural, and society has pushed the shame onto you.

However, you do not need to live there. You are a human being. You have rights because you exist. You legally deserve equal treatment, even if you don't always get it. And you can still have a great life despite these challenges.

You can navigate the broken systems we face: Reinforcing your ability to recognize and work through ableism

It isn't our fault that we're disabled. It isn't our fault that structural ableism exists. It isn't our fault that society is penalizing us for aspects of our identity they don't understand.

Not being at fault doesn't mean we bear no responsibility for our actions or the impacts society has on us. I don't approve of "playing the victim" or otherwise allowing this brokenness to run our lives. We are fighting an uphill battle against a system that is biased against us. That doesn't mean we give up.

It means it's time for us to manage our expectations, recognize the full challenges we face, and plan ahead so we can still succeed despite these obstacles. We do all that while managing our conditions. This isn't easy, but it is necessary.

As disabled people, we face extra stresses, more chances of social exclusion, and a higher risk of being abused, neglected, or considered incompetent than abled people.

Like any minority identity, disabled folks are identified as "other" and given extra hoops to jump through. As always, the more minority identities you have, the more likely you are to be given a hard time based on any of your identities.

This absolutely isn't fair. It isn't just. It isn't equitable. But it is our current reality. And facing that reality is the only way to get through while protecting your mental and emotional health.

With each step in the processes in these books, take time to remind yourself most of the obstacles and difficulties in your way are the result of some form of bias other people have (or that you've been taught by society to carry).

The challenge is not your fault or failure, but a symptom of a broken system that is rigged against you. You still need to take the steps to get the thing you need, but it isn't personal, it isn't something you did wrong. It simply is.

While you absolutely deserve better, better may not be on the menu at the moment. You still need that support, service, or opportunity, so you still need to jump through those hoops. And you still won't get the thing until the gatekeepers let you through.

Know that this is because they are participating in a biased system, not because of any fault or failure on your part. You need to game the system for your survival, because you need to take care of yourself. It is your responsibility to take care of you, because nobody else knows what you need better.

You deserve enough food to eat, a safe place to live, the medical care you need for a good quality of life, and to spend time with people who love you and want you to be happy. It shouldn't be too much to ask. However, societal messaging may well suggest otherwise.

I want you to know that you do deserve all these things, and that many of the challenges along the way are the result of structural ableism (and/or other societal biases). Each step you take in getting yourself the care you need, and in creating or maintaining healthy relationships is another step from surviving your disability to thriving as a person with a disability.

KEY POINTS

- **Universal benefits of Social Welfare:** Despite the stigma, everyone benefits from social welfare supports, whether through direct assistance or broader societal improvements.
- **Navigating the Broken System:** Despite the brokenness of the system, it is possible to navigate these challenges and advocate for the support and resources needed to improve your quality of life.

RESOURCES

Government Programs

Office of Family Assistance: "Temporary Assistance for Needy Families (TANF)." Accessed July 8, 2024: **https://www.acf.hhs.gov/ofa/programs/tanf**.

Internal Revenue Service: "Don't Forget, Social Security Benefits May Be Taxable." Accessed July 8, 2024: **https://www.irs.gov/newsroom/dont-forget-social-security-benefits-may-be-taxable**.

The other listed programs are discussed in detail in Volume II.

RESOURCES WEBPAGE » CHAPTER 5

CHAPTER 6

Social Realities of Disability

How and why your web of social support may fray when you become disabled

Relationships are all exchanges of energy. While there is recognition that becoming disabled is financially expensive (medical bills and lost wages), it's also socially and emotionally expensive.

It is terrifyingly easy to become socially isolated after a serious injury or illness. Ableism plays a large part, but it goes even deeper than that. I'll use the term "friends" throughout this section, but similar things can happen within your family or to your romantic relationships.

I'm specifically focused on the losses you might experience, why they may happen, and what you may be able to do to minimize the damage. Friendships and social interactions are vital for everyone's mental health, so maintaining connections with others is a very important part of your healing process. If that is not possible, building new social connections becomes even more important.

Having a chronic or severe illness or injury is pretty much guaranteed to break up most of the patterns and cycles in your life, including disrupting those patterns with friends. These disruptions have the potential to ruin friendships, redefine relationships, and lead to you feeling isolated and alone.

They can shake up your relationships, potentially increasing how connected you feel with some friends, and showing you how important you and your friendship is to others.

Your actions and decisions, and those of your friends, will determine how your life is affected. Let's try to keep those changes as positive as possible, okay?

Social Signatures: Human limitations in friendship, and how that is affected by a disabling condition

A study[25] from 2014 indicates that each person has their own "social signature." The social signature is simply an indicator of the number of close relationships a person has, as compared to their list of social acquaintances.

The almost universal trait identified in the study is that participants (and presumably most, if not all, people) had more social acquaintances than close friends. The interesting part is that each person in the study had a consistent number of "close friends" with whom they communicated regularly and intensely.

Who those friends were changed over time, with some dropping out of the picture (losing the friendship), and some shifting to a more distant relationship (becoming social acquaintances), but each person consistently had the same number of close friends.

Later in the article, the author speaks about three constraints on each person's social signature, and how consistent each person's social signature was:

1. **Time:** No matter what, there are only 24 hours in the day, and there is a limit to how much of that time we have to focus on our friends, as opposed to working, sleeping, and so on.

2. **Emotional capital/energy:** Creating and maintaining friendships takes emotional energy. We only have so much emotional energy to invest in our friendships—and changing that amount of emotional energy would require a large change in lifestyle, if it is even possible.

---

25 Huffington Post: "Science May Explain Why Your Friendships Fall Apart" blog post; webpage: **https://www.huffpost.com/entry/social-signature-friends_b_4590203**

3. **Cognitive/mental capacity:** Our brains don't have the capability to handle an infinite number of social connections, so at some point, we aren't capable of adding more friends.

When we experience a big physical or emotional trauma (such as a severe injury or a chronic condition getting worse), it takes a lot of emotional energy to process, leaving less energy available for growing or maintaining friendships.

These traumas are going to abruptly disrupt most of the patterns and schedules in your life, which means your availability will change—and the old patterns you and your friends were used to get disrupted.

While it's possible you will end up with more time available, it's less likely to be the same time as your friends. With lowered emotional energy, extra time being devoted to resting and healing, and many of your life patterns interrupted, it's very difficult to maintain your social signature.

Even if you can maintain multiple friendships, you likely don't have the bandwidth for as many close friends as you used to. That's a loss you may feel for the rest of your life.

Friendships and FND—becoming disabled in my early 20's

I had my first FND symptoms while I was in college. My friends mostly supported me and helped me get to a neurologist and get treatment.

There was no real diagnosis at the time (a vague "It's anxiety, take these pills, they might help," was all I was told). I was in a very anxious headspace and leaned on my friends at college for support.

The symptoms decreased dramatically in a few weeks and, within a month or so, they seemed completely gone.

I made several decisions that effectively relegated most of my friends to the "social acquaintances" identity in the years that followed. During my senior year of college, I spent two of my three terms off-campus, with a semester in Woods Hole, MA, studying saltwater and terrestrial ecosystems, and then my winter term in London, where I completed my fine arts requirement. Both experiences were wonderful, but at each location I only had one person I knew well sharing each experience with me. I returned to campus for my final term and reconnected with friends, but we all knew we only had a few months until graduation.

After graduation, I spent about six months back at home in New Jersey, where I reconnected with friends from before college, some of whom had stayed in the area. Then I was off again, and spent about 8 months traveling in Australia, then spent a month in the UK. Shortly after my return to New Jersey, I accepted a position as a fishery observer in the Gulf of Mexico, and so was off again, flying to Texas for training, then going out to sea for my first trip. After I returned home, a friend and I decided to rent an apartment together, but things fell apart when I got back from my second trip. It turned out the position had lost funding, so I no longer had a job, and it was now mid-December so there likely wouldn't be openings in my field for at least the next several months.

My friends from college were scattered around the country, but nobody I was close to settled anywhere near me (this wasn't a huge surprise, as I'd gone to college in the Midwest), and my friends from before college had gotten pretty used to me being absent. My friend who became a roommate and I did move in together, and our apartment became the central location for gatherings with the two other friends who had stayed or returned to New Jersey.

The stress of losing that job, and the uncertainty that surrounded it (they kept hoping to cobble together financial support to keep things going, and I didn't think to apply for unemployment benefits), triggered the return of my movement symptoms and increasing urinary urgency symptoms.

Besides the four of us having known one another for years, they had known me through a few depressive episodes, a brief period of self-cutting, my uncle's death by suicide, and my choir director's death from a heart attack. All three of these friends who remained in New Jersey had lost a parent since I'd met them. We had all been through emotional trauma and grief, and I had been supportive of them through their processes, and they had been supportive of me through mine.

These were friendships that had already been tested and had made the cut. That, I think, is why I didn't have a severe loss of friends when my FND kicked in. However, it is likely that if my FND hadn't kicked in, I would have been actively searching for additional potential friends.

I spent about six months trying to get diagnosed. My friends in New Jersey had brought me back into their "close friend" slots. I think it helped that my roommate and I were the only ones in our groups of friends who weren't living with our parents, so our place was the obvious location for any get-together.

The other thing I think really helped, was that I was willing to talk to them about what was happening—our friendships had already survived an unusual amount of trauma for our ages.

I clearly communicated what I knew about both the urgency and the movements and kept them posted on appointments and what I learned in them. I did my best to make sure that I asked my friends how they were doing and what was happening in their lives, so they knew that I cared. I worked hard to not make my health stuff the center of our conversations.

My health issues would center some of my one-on-one conversations, but in group conversations I tried to stay focused on enjoying my friends and being part of the discussion.

It helped that they were very considerate of my needs, so we were all happy to do a lot of things in our apartment or, if we went out, to go somewhere with an easily accessible bathroom and any other support I needed.

Because those lines of communication were so open, it was easier after my FND diagnosis to discuss what else was happening. I still felt a bit lonely, but that made sense, too, with all I was dealing with (especially the depression), and my "close friend" pool wasn't as full as it normally would have been. In the terms used by the study, I had fewer people filling my "close friend" slots than my social signature normally would have suggested. I did not have the energy to try to fill it more.

In the years since, my energy levels have varied, with periods of doing well and periods of relapse or major traumas. I have connected with a lot of people over the years, but I think we tended to mutually be in more of a social acquaintance category most of the time. The exceptions have been friendships that turned into dating relationships. However, I've learned to cherish the connections I have, and enjoy them for what they are. The nice part is, whenever I have the energy, I have a list of people I'd like to catch up with, and usually one or more of them are happy to reconnect and make plans.

Recognizing that friendships go both ways

Friendships are always a mutual decision, where both or all people involved have actively decided that they care about one another and want to both provide and receive help from one another.

Each person only has the mental, emotional, and structural capacity to have so many friends, and injury or illness is likely to reduce your mental and emotional capacity to focus on your friends and maintain those friendships.

In some cases that damage is long-term or permanent (with most chronic conditions, things can improve or worsen, but you might never return to the full capacity you had before your condition began), while in other cases the damage might be more temporary (a serious but short-term illness might only put you out of commission for a few days or weeks. A break, fracture, or other injuries may be debilitating at first, but you recover over time, allowing your energy levels to bounce back).

Either way, the patterns you have developed with your friends will be disrupted, and you will either make decisions that help your friendships survive your trauma or make decisions that don't help keep your friendships alive.

Even though you did not intentionally step away from the friendship due to your condition, it may (subconsciously) feel that way to your friend—after all, they didn't do anything that would cause a change to the relationship.

Your best step is maintaining open communication with your friends and, if that feels too overwhelming, trusting your gut and sharing the information with the friends you can.

Recognize that losing a friendship may very well have nothing to do with you or your choices. In many cases, witnessing someone you care about having a health crisis, trauma, or major life pattern disruption can be very stressful. Your friend may not have the mental or emotional bandwidth to deal with your situation, or it may trigger their own fears, traumatic memories, or other stressors. If they see something is wrong and you're not sharing information with them, they may feel that you don't value their friendship.

As we've discussed before, our society has many ableist biases, and your friends may simply be unwilling or unable to understand your new situation and support you through those changes.

While there is no healthy long-term way for you to ignore your disability, all your friend needs to do is allow you to drop out of their life, and they won't need to think about your disability (or their mortality) anymore. This may not be the healthiest decision in the long run, but it certainly isn't a severely damaging one for them.

You are likely to lose some friends through the process of becoming disabled (or recognizing that you are), and very often that is more a commentary on them than it is on you.

For the friendships you are most concerned about protecting, you may want to plan out conversational time with those friends individually.

Preparing for friendship and disability conversations

1. **Know what or how much you are comfortable telling this friend about your current issue.** Your job is to bridge the gap in their knowledge or experience, so you can truly communicate again. You can explain things like their risk of catching your condition (usually non-existent), what you are feeling, physically or emotionally, and what effects your condition has on your day-to-day existence. If you know you are already dealing with misunderstandings or frustrations, do your best to explain how or why these things happened and how you hope to avoid them happening again. You do not need to blame yourself or fall on your sword, but you do want to be clear, honest, and non-accusatory (in other words, this situation is nobody's FAULT, just the natural result of events beyond anyone's control).

2. **Have one or two very specific requests, things they can do to help you through your situation.** The nature of that request depends on what's happening, but things like scheduling time to talk, being understanding if you don't respond quickly, or advocating with your friends and/or family for quieter or closer activities would all be good examples. The point is it should be a very identifiable thing that you know will help you, and something concrete they will likely be able and willing to do once asked. You shouldn't ask them to move mountains, but instead to help clear your path.

3. **Make your plans for a day, time, and location that is comfortable for both of you, and that will give you the privacy (and/or anonymity) to have this conversation without interruption.** This might be your house, or theirs, or a nearby coffee shop or park. Wherever you meet, make sure you will not be rushed or interrupted and you both feel comfortable there. Both of you are likely under enough stress as it is, and meeting in a safe space will help you both focus on the conversation.

4. **Plan when and how you are going to start the conversation.** If you are anxious, this is especially important. A conversation like this is displaying vulnerability and a lot of us have a hard time with that. So have a plan for starting the conversation. It can be "I'll start right after we order our coffee" or "She needs to vent about her family for a bit, so I'll ask her how she's doing, and then share when she asks how I am." Whatever you need, do it, but be sure to give yourself a firm plan about when and how you are going to start the conversation.

5. **Carry through.** Make your plans with your friend and, if it feels appropriate, let them know you have something you want to talk about when you make plans. Some people appreciate a heads up that you might have an intense conversation or that you have a specific thing you want to discuss. Other friends might interpret a statement of "we have to talk" as something threatening or anxiety producing. Think about your friend's needs and interpretation of your request and then act appropriately. You want them to be in the best possible state of mind to have an open and intimate conversation.

6. **Make space for your friend to share concerns, respond, or otherwise give you feedback.** This needs to be a conversation, not a set of statements. While telling your friend what is happening to you and what support you need, make sure that your friend knows you are sharing this because you trust them and because you value their friendship and insight. This confirms to them they are valuable and important to you and you are concerned about preserving your friendship with them.

7. **If all goes well, recruit them to help you strategize who else to talk to and when.** Your friend can be a great source of insight and feedback about how, as a friend, your changes are being interpreted. They are the best person to help you make sure the message gets expressed clearly to mutual friends or challenging family members. This friend can help make the explanation process go easier and potentially help other members of your circle of friends understand better.

These conversations may not save all your friendships, but they will help you keep and strengthen the friendships that are most likely to survive your situation. Among other things, a willingness to have this conversation indicates their openness to saving or protecting the friendship!

Social risks due to disability

Having a disability increases your risk of social isolation. It can increase your risks of divorce[26] (if married) or of abuse[27] in general. Let's talk about these risks so that you understand why that's the case and can protect yourself should the worst happen.

As always, I'm trying to help you protect yourself and to understand, should you find yourself in this position, you are far from alone, and you should not shoulder all (likely any) of the blame for it.

 GLOBAL

The risks I discuss may very well be universal, but the details of how it impacts your finances and what legal protections you have and need, will vary by country. Use this information to guide your searches, but if you live outside of the US, please explore your local laws and protections and don't assume they are the same as they are in the US!

Divorce risk

Whenever one member of a couple experiences a trauma, both partners are impacted. When a partner becomes disabled, especially permanently, this increases the pressure on both partners in different ways. We've talked about how, as the disabled partner, you're likely to experience shame and a sense of failure and may feel like a burden, but the pressures on the abled partner can also be quite intense.

---

26 Insult to Injury: Disability, Earnings, and Divorce, by Perry Singleton: **https://www.researchgate.net/publication/46435226_Insult_to_Injury_Disability_Earnings_and_Divorce**

27 "Victims with Disabilities," Office for Victims of Crime, Office of Justice Programs, U.S. Department of Justice, accessed April 10, 2025, **https://ovc.ojp.gov/topics/victims-with-disabilities**.

For them, they are facing much darker financial prospects than expected and can opt out by leaving. They may be experiencing social pressure to exit the relationship as disabled people are, all too often, written off by society. On top of all that, they may be in the unexpected position of becoming your caregiver, which can be exhausting and may lead to emotional burnout.

All of these are explanations, not excuses. The article "Insult to Injury" (in the resources section) discusses how the biggest indicators for divorce are the age of the disabled individual and the severity of the disability. The identity group most likely to get divorced are younger, educated men who become disabled, as they were socially expected to provide the lion's share of the earnings and financial support within the relationship. Couples where one member becomes permanently disabled are more likely than not to end up divorcing.

Disability has the greatest impact on marriage when a couple has a disabled child (up to 87% of couples with a "severely disabled" child divorce[28]), though that may partially be the result of the brokenness of our social welfare system, as children only get SSI coverage (and in some cases Medicaid) if their household is low income. Divorcing often lowers household income, especially if one of the parents becomes primary caregiver and has to reduce work hours or stop working altogether.

What I'm saying here is that disability can greatly increase the risk of divorce. If you are facing this situation, know that you are far from alone. You need to understand that, if your spouse can't handle you becoming disabled, in the long term divorce is likely better for you, emotionally, than staying in the marriage and trying to mask your disability. That's not going to make it hurt any less, but it is worth recognizing.

If you are looking at the possibility of a divorce, make sure you are as protected as possible. You should have a divorce attorney, preferably one with experience with disability-related laws and considerations (there is an organization for that purpose, the Special Needs Alliance, listed in resources below), and you should know what rules you need to follow to get the benefits you will need to survive.

---

28 Ann Gold Buscho, "Divorce and Special Needs Children," Psychology Today, February 16, 2023, **https://www.psychologytoday.com/us/blog/a-better-divorce/202302/divorce-and-special-needs-children**.

Basically, before you agree on an amount of alimony or other financial support, make sure you understand the rules for your state (or country), so you become or remain eligible for the programs you need. If you and your spouse co-own a house, you may want to evaluate if that house makes sense for you in the long term, and if it's something you want to fight for. Divorces often lead to a couple selling their home to divide the financial value, with the alternative being one spouse buying the other spouse out. However, other solutions can sometimes be negotiated if both parties agree.

Depending on your situation, this may be your best (or only) opportunity for home ownership. If you do co-own a house, it may be a space that will no longer meet your needs, so you may be the one pushing to sell the home or be bought out.

Only you can decide what your priorities are, but I want to encourage you to consider all of this from the disability angle—both in the sense of what's best for you physically and emotionally, and what's most useful for you financially. You deserve to be in the best possible situation on all fronts, and knowing the rules before sitting down to negotiate will help you come out of the divorce in the best possible position for your long-term financial, physical, and emotional health.

Physical or emotional abuse risk

You are at a higher risk of abuse. Like any minority identity (we'll discuss this in the next section), you are now easier to victimize and less likely to be believed. Being socially isolated increases your chances of missing warning signs of potential abusers and having fewer friends to help you recognize standard patterns of long-term abusers. Being aware of this may help you protect yourself.

While abuse is most prevalent with people with intellectual or developmental disabilities[29,] we all should be and stay aware of these risks.

As a woman, I've been trained to be on guard against certain risks, like rape in all its forms (date rape, random street attacks, etc.). As a disabled woman, I know I'm at higher risk than abled women for any of these to occur.

---

29 "Abuse and Exploitation," Disability Justice, accessed April 10, 2025, **https://disabilityjustice.org/justice-denied/abuse-and-exploitation/**.

Disabled people are more than twice as likely (2.5 times)[30] to be victims of non-fatal violent crimes as abled people in non-institutional settings (meaning this is not taking into account the folks who are institutionalized).

We are more likely to be bullied, raped, and otherwise attacked than abled folks. We are at greater risk of being injured or killed by police[31] than abled folks.

This is especially true when we are part of another marginalized identity (such as being a person of color, part of the LGBT+ community, etc.) and/or have a disability that's especially likely to be subject to prejudice (e.g., a deaf person not responding to verbal warnings, or having a mental illness, challenges in communicating, or an intellectual disability).

How can you protect yourself? The first step is awareness. Knowing you look like a potential target can help you be prepared to navigate challenging situations (or avoid them altogether). Staying financially independent can be very helpful too, as being in control of your own money makes it easier for you to leave a situation that turns abusive.

Be careful about sharing identifying information in open forums or to interested individuals. Don't give people money or ways to get money from you. You don't need to be hyper-suspicious but think about why somebody might want to know something before volunteering information. Understand your rights, don't accept what random people tell you.

There is a greater risk of being abused by your family and friends. If you are part of a dysfunctional family, you may have already experienced some of this, and may already be thinking about it, but disability may make things even more complicated.

---

30 Erica L. Smith and Rachel E. Morgan, Crime Against Persons with Disabilities, 2009-2015 - Statistical Tables (Washington, DC: Bureau of Justice Statistics, 2017), **https://bjs.ojp.gov/library/publications/crime-against-persons-disabilities-2009-2015-statistical-tables**.

31 Antonia Hylton and Andrew Blankstein, "Half of People Killed by Police Suffer from Mental Disability: Report," NBC News, March 1, 2016, **https://www.nbcnews.com/news/us-news/half-people-killed-police-suffer-mental-disability-report-n538371**.

Because ableism is so pervasive, there's a good chance some of your family and friends (if not most) will have some form of ableist bent. This may be as simple as discouraging you from applying for disability (even if you should) to berating you for your "laziness" or assuming your symptoms are actions you've chosen to take.

You may be accused of lying or exaggerating, or you may have family members decide to cut you out of family events or communications or otherwise pretend you don't exist.

I am not trying to scare you with these possibilities, nor am I telling you to actively distrust people. What I am saying is to take some time to observe when, how, and why the people closest to you help out, and to consider your history with them before making any major decisions or giving anyone any special power over you or your money.

It's already hard enough living with a disability. The brokenness of the social welfare system already makes things hard, leaves you vulnerable, and puts you in a tough situation. Don't let yourself fall into additional traps by putting your trust in somebody who will abuse it. You deserve to be treated fairly, so be sure to protect yourself.

There are many red flags to watch out for, and many forms of abuse to consider, but at its most basic, you want to feel confident the people you trust truly want you to succeed and have your best interests at heart.

If you frequently find yourself feeling guilty, uncertain, or frightened around someone, pause and consider why. If you tend to feel worse about yourself when around them, pause and consider why. If other friends or family who you trust warn you away from this specific person, consider why, and who has what to gain from it.

No one can truly thrive completely on their own. We humans are very social creatures. But you do want to be and remain as independent as possible, and anyone who seems to be making that harder, or leaves you feeling bad for trying to create or maintain that independence deserves to get a bit of a side eye.

Financial Abuse or Neglect Risk

If an individual has trouble managing money but can take care of their daily living, they may want or need a representative payee. This is a designated person who can handle financial transactions and who collects the disabled individual's checks.

In many cases, a parent is a representative payee, but that is not legally required. In fact, adults generally select their own representative payee, which is useful in most cases, but can lead to abuse if a person isn't careful about it.

There is a risk of someone demanding to become your representative payee or trying to have you declared incompetent so they can manage your money or property.

If you or a family member are at risk (or in need) of having a representative payee, guardian, or other legally recognized mediator of your life decisions, be sure that much consideration is given to the least invasive ways to provide those supports, and what protections are in place to minimize the risk of abuse.

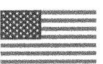 **UNITED STATES OF AMERICA**

You can select a representative payee in advance if you are on SSDI or SSI, so that should you become unable to manage your money, somebody is already in place to do so. Protect yourself or your family member by making sure that:

1. A representative payee is only designated if truly necessary, and
2. The person designated will be making decisions with the disabled individual's best interests at heart, and where possible, with the disabled person's input.

Most disabled people do not need a legal guardian or to otherwise be treated as sub-adult once they reach adulthood. However, there are cases where people really do need these supports. Some disabled people do need a legal guardian after they become an adult, post-injury, or as they age, but others can have Supported Decision-Making put in place instead.

Basically, Supported Decision-Making gives others some aspects of guardianship, but provides additional protections to the disabled individual so the risk of being forced into an untenable situation is reduced and their desires are more likely to receive legal protections. The exact laws and protections will vary by state, but if you or a family member are facing these concerns, it's well worth researching (links in the resources section below).

For too many disabled people who cannot direct their own care (make decisions for their financial and physical wellbeing) or who are presumed not to be able to, they may be institutionalized in the least expensive (and/or easiest) way possible without consideration for their individual need or desires. These sorts of decisions increase their odds of being physically or emotionally abused or neglected in the places providing them with long-term care[32].

I want to be very clear on this: if you cannot do your activities of daily living but are mentally capable of directing your care (communicating your needs and desires to others), you do not need the sort of care discussed here, but instead should be eligible for Home and Community Based Care supports through Medicaid (discussed in Volume II), or similar programs. Supported Decision-Making, institutionalization, and related concepts are for people who cannot or will not be able to reliably make sound financial and/or care decisions, not people who are temporarily challenged or who are managing purely (or primarily) physical limitations. It is very difficult to undo or cancel legal guardianship, so please explore other options and view guardianship as the nuclear option that it is.

Family decision-making about a disabled person's options

When your family is already struggling, all the challenges discussed above can be made worse. Keeping a severely disabled family member at home can be overwhelming to any family, especially a medically complex family member who needs support 24/7 when the family is not equipped to do so. There's potential for abuse or neglect from family members, which can be very damaging to the disabled individual.

---

[32] National Center on Elder Abuse, Research Brief: Maltreatment of Adults in Long-Term Care Settings (Washington, DC: National Center on Elder Abuse, 2016), **https://www.centeronelderabuse.org/docs/ResearchBrief_LongTermCare_508web.pdf**.

There is no single right solution to most disability-related challenges, rather there are a variety of better and worse options somebody needs to think through. Ideally, the best person to make the decision is the individual with the disability, but this is not always possible.

If you may be facing these sorts of challenges, do your best to protect yourself by ensuring your desires are recorded somewhere (such as a living will) and/or if you know specific family members or friends really understand your perspective, you create legal documents (like Durable Power of Attorney) that put those responsibilities on them. These processes are discussed in more detail in Volume II in the Marriage chapter.

There are situations where being institutionalized or placed into supportive housing (discussed in Volume II) is the best possible option, and only the disabled individual and their family are best placed to determine that. Institutional situations vary widely, some are high-quality, others are not. Some spaces can be nurturing and supportive, but too many are underfunded or run by a corporation focused on reducing costs rather than improving client satisfaction, which can lead to neglect and increase the risk of abuse.

Understaffing and high staff turnover commonly accompany these issues and increase the risk of individuals being abused or neglected. With Covid-19, way too many elderly and disabled people died due to living in communal settings (residents and staff of long-term care facilities were 22% of Covid-19 fatalities while making up about 2% of the population)[33].

No matter the situation, family members are usually the people determining where the person with these types of disabilities ends up living. Making decisions that are in that person's best interest is important, while wherever possible taking their desires into consideration and involving them in these decisions to the best of their ability.

If you or a friend or family member is facing the possibility of needing institutionalization or being unable to make long term financial or self-care decisions, take the time to consider the options and recognize the challenges, so that you (or they) can plan the best possible long-term solution.

---

33   Elizabeth Hinton and Cornelia Hall, "10 Things About Long-Term Services and Supports (LTSS)," KFF, October 26, 2023, **https://www.kff.org/medicaid/issue-brief/10-things-about-long-term-services-and-supports-ltss/**.

This may include designating a representative payee (I already have designated Al as mine, in case any form of accident occurs to cause these challenges), researching local supportive housing options (discussed in the housing section in Volume II), or having conversations about these possibilities with friends or family members. If your condition is likely to cause limitations in your ability to communicate or make decisions, protect yourself now, while you still have the capacity. If a friend or relative is already in this type of situation, you may be able to guide them (or their more immediate family members) towards solutions that are respectful and supportive.

KEY POINTS

- **Disabled people are at higher risk of abuse and neglect than abled people.**
- **Your social support network** (friendships and familial relationships) may weaken because of life changes and decreased energy associated with disability.
- Taking **proactive steps** like planned conversations with friends can help mitigate these changes, ensuring support and inclusion.
- It is important to be cautious, especially with **financial dependence**, as disability can increase the risk of divorce (if married) and of abuse.
- Some people with disabilities may need a designated representative payee or supportive decision-making put in place if they are unable to make significant decisions about their finances or care.
- Legal guardianship leaves the disabled individual legally sub-adult the rest of their life, so it should only be the last resort if a person is never going to recover.

RESOURCES

Social Losses due to Disability

Thriving While Disabled: "Disability and Loneliness" blog post; webpage: **https://thrivingwhiledisabled.com/disability-and-loneliness/**

Thriving While Disabled: "Losing friends due to chronic illness" blog post; webpage: **https://thrivingwhiledisabled.com/losing-friends-due-to-chronic-illness/**

Thriving While Disabled: "Why Friendships Fall Apart After Severe Illness or Injury" blog post; webpage: **https://thrivingwhiledisabled.com/why-friendships-fall-apart/**

Disability and Divorce

"Disability Leads to Divorce? The Data Is Daunting." People's Problems. Accessed April 10, 2025. **https://www.peoplesproblems.org/showblog/288/disability-leads-to-divorce-the-data-is-daunting**.

Anderson, Kari. "Divorce and Special Needs Children." Psychology Today, February 28, 2023. **https://www.psychologytoday.com/us/blog/a-better-divorce/202302/divorce-and-special-needs-children**.

Hughes, Barbara, and Edward V. Wilcenski. "When People with Disabilities Divorce." Special Needs Alliance, December 12, 2024. **https://www.specialneedsalliance.org/blog/when-people-with-disabilities-divorce/**.

Disability and Abuse

"Abuse and Exploitation." Disability Justice. Accessed April 10, 2025. **https://disabilityjustice.org/justice-denied/abuse-and-exploitation/**.

"Victims with Disabilities." Office for Victims of Crime, Office of Justice Programs. Accessed April 10, 2025. **https://ovc.ojp.gov/topics/victims-with-disabilities**.

Long Term Care Facilities and Risk of Abuse

National Research Council (US) Panel to Review Risk and Prevalence of Elder Abuse and Neglect; Bonnie RJ, Wallace RB, editors.Washington (DC): National Academies Press (US); 2003. **https://www.ncbi.nlm.nih.gov/books/NBK98786/**

Administration for Community Living. "Protecting Rights & Preventing Abuse." Administration for Community Living, last updated February 29, 2024. **https://acl.gov/programs/protecting-rights-and-preventing-abuse**.

Supported Decision Making

National Resource Center for Supported Decision-Making. "Supported Decision-Making." Supported Decision-Making, 2024. **https://supporteddecisionmaking.org/**.

ACLU. "FAQ About Supported Decision-Making." American Civil Liberties Union, last updated February 2016. **https://www.aclu.org/sites/default/files/field_document/faq_about_supported_decision_making.pdf**.

RESOURCES WEBPAGE » CHAPTER 6

CHAPTER 7

Minority Stress
Disability counts too!

The Stress of having a Minority Identity

Many scientists argue that simply having a stigmatized identity in modern society is stressful in and of itself. This designation, "minority stress", covers not only racial minorities (like Black people, Asians, Native Americans, or Hispanics), but other minority identities, such as the LGBT community.

While minority stress was initially explored as a model covering non-heterosexual orientations, it has been applied to other communities as well, including women, religious minorities, racial minorities, and more.

I have absolutely experienced minority stress; the type and severity have varied dramatically.

A brief example of experiencing being a racial minority was the time I went with my Hispanic partner and his parents to a Hispanic grocery store a few towns away. Wandering through the store with them, I suddenly realized that I was the lightest-skinned person in the store (just by a shade or two, but still…), and the only one who didn't speak Spanish. I had a moment of my mind being blown and I remembered realizing "THIS is what they were talking about in class, the stress of simply knowing there's nobody else like you around."

I immediately saw the unspoken pressure of simply being different from everyone around you. Nobody did anything to make me feel unwelcome, and I was with people whom I loved and trusted, and I still had that extreme moment of recognition that I am "other" from the group around me. It's an uncomfortable feeling, and one I still have difficulty imagining as a consistent, daily feeling, though I'm very aware this is the reality for many people (including racial minorities and people with visible disabilities). It's something I hadn't recognized experiencing before, but the emotional aspect is something I've recognized many times since.

> **Most of my disability-related minority stress experiences have been inextricably tied to overt ableism to some degree or other.**
>
> There was the time on the train when a conductor saw me rocking back and forth (I had a long day, including two grad school classes) and quietly asked everyone around me if they were traveling with me because 1) She assumed I was incapable of traveling by myself, and 2) She was concerned that I was going to injure myself with my rocking motion.
>
> When I realized the first part of what she was doing, I stopped rocking (this was enough of a distraction) and asked her if she had a question for me. Startled (and possibly a little guilty at realizing that I wasn't incapable of communication), she stammered out concern that I might injure myself and asked if I shouldn't wait before riding the train.
>
> Later, I realized the perfect comeback would have been "How should I get home then? Drive?", but at the time I was angry and embarrassed and likely just said that I would be okay. The ableism was her presumptions, the internalized ableism was my embarrassment over doing what my body needed to do, and the anger was a response to the whole stressful situation that wouldn't have occurred if ableism didn't exist. All of it together is the minority stress in response to bias.

> I have had so many times that I've been aware of people staring at me when I've been badly symptomatic, asking what was wrong with my leg when they saw me limping (nothing, my brain's just sending bad signals to it), pushing me to get in a wheelchair, stop participating, or go home the moment I had symptoms, or otherwise signaling to me that I was other, different, or less valuable due to their interpretation of my symptoms.

These actions implied that I was unaware of these things, or incapable of making good decisions due to having a disability. Whether ignorantly ableist or spoken with the best of intentions by people who love me, these are all examples of stresses I have experienced due to my minority identity as a person with a disability. A useful term for most of these behaviors is microaggressions[34], which is most easily explained as a slight (verbal or nonverbal) that impacts an individual from a marginalized or non-mainstream community.

The disabled identity is a minority identity

Disabled people are the largest minority identity in the US, covering about 27% of the US population[35]. This covers a very broad definition of disability and a very wide range of symptoms and limitations.

We experience minority stress, plus the individual challenges that our disabilities (and society's lack of accessibility) create. That's a lot of chronic stress to manage.

Not only that, but many of us with disabilities have intersectional minority identities as well. The disability community is extremely diverse and the only minority identity that any person can end up joining at any point in their lives.

---

34 "Microaggression," Psychology Today, accessed April 10, 2025, **https://www.psychologytoday.com/us/basics/microaggression**.
35 "Disability Impacts All of Us," Centers for Disease Control and Prevention, last reviewed March 2, 2023, **https://www.cdc.gov/ncbddd/disabilityandhealth/infographic-disability-impacts-all.html**.

So, for those of us who are disabled, we're managing the stress of our conditions (chronic illness being recognized as one of the biggest situational stresses out there), the stress of societal response to our being disabled, and the stresses that most folks who share other aspects of our particular identity share with us.

As an example, I am a poor disabled bisexual cis-gendered white woman. I'm managing the stresses of FND (a stress-responsive neurological condition that's poorly understood), migraines, a history of mental illness (and the stigma that goes with that), the stress of being openly bisexual (less stressful than trying to pass as straight), the stress associated with classism, and the stress of being a woman in a sexist society.

There's a lot to unpack, but my point is that there are a lot of aspects of who I am that expose me to extra stresses.

Is it any wonder that my immune system seems weaker than average?

Having multiple stress-responsive conditions means the better I manage my mindset, and the more successful I am at managing my stresses, the more likely I am to have a better-quality life.

Managing stress as a minority identity

I want to help you be aware you aren't imagining that life is harder for you than for the average person—it really is. The first thing I hope you do with this data is to absorb what it means—you really are dealing with a lot of external stress and pressure.

Those pressures may increase your risk of complications and make it easier to trigger some, if not all, of your symptoms. You are at a higher risk of internalizing those pressures, being even more self-critical than you might otherwise be.

That's the bad news.

The good news is that you aren't alone.

While you likely have one or more minority identities, the work you do to help yourself manage stress should help you manage many of these pressures. Finding others like you can help you feel more understood, but people don't need to share all qualities with you to be able to empathize with your challenges.

The skills associated with stress management are similar across the board. Taking time to journal, for example, will help you process your challenges as a whole being, however many minority identities you have. The same goes for meditation (which we'll discuss later in Chapter 10), mindfulness, listening to your body, taking naps, and many other aspects of self-care and stress management. Knowing the tendencies of those who share your identity may help you recognize the risks you are particularly predisposed towards and manage them.

Turning to any form of addictive substance or behavior, as an example, is a risk for people managing stress, as it relieves the pressure temporarily but is likely to cause health issues in the long term. Recognizing that risk may help you moderate activities that frequently become addictive.

Personally, my awareness of my family's history of alcohol addiction, for example, keeps me aware of if and how often I consume alcohol. That doesn't mean I don't drink it, but I do actively avoid developing habits involving alcohol consumption—and I make a point of not drinking if I am in a position of emotional instability. In other words, I'll happily have a drink with friends to enhance my enjoyment, but I'm not going to drink to escape my stresses.

Being a minority is stressful, especially with all the bias expressed out in the world. Being disabled is a minority identity, and subject to those same pressures. Recognizing these pressures are out there can help you better recognize the associated stresses and manage them, including giving yourself a break.

Ableism is as real as racism and sexism, and all too often we have absorbed aspects of those attitudes as well.

How do you manage your minority stress? By recognizing its reality and finding ways to reaffirm your value to yourself.

Now that you're aware of the legitimacy of your identity as a person with a disability, make sure you care for yourself, including being kind to yourself about each step of your journey.

Recognizing the minority stresses you face doesn't make them go away, but that recognition can help you find the solutions you need to these challenges.

KEY POINTS

- About 27% of Americans have a disability, making it the **largest minority identity** in the country.
- As a minority identity, people with disabilities experience **minority stress** and its associated challenges.

RESOURCES

Minority Stress

"What is Minority Stress?," University of Rochester Medical Center, published in 2025, **https://www.urccp.org/article.cfm?ArticleNumber=69**.

Ilan H. Meyer, "Prejudice, Social Stress, and Mental Health in Lesbian, Gay, and Bisexual Populations: Conceptual Issues and Research Evidence," Psychological Bulletin 129, no. 5 (2003): 674–97. **https://pubmed.ncbi.nlm.nih.gov/12956539/**

Emily M. Lund, "Examining the potential applicability of the minority stress model for explaining suicidality in individuals with disabilities," Rehabilitation Psychology 66, no. 3 (May 2021): 233–43. **https://pubmed.ncbi.nlm.nih.gov/34014712/**

Suzanne C. Segerstrom and Gregory E. Miller, "Psychological Stress and the Human Immune System: A Meta-Analytic Study of 30 Years of Inquiry," Psychological Bulletin 130, no. 4 (July 2004): 601–30. **https://pubmed.ncbi.nlm.nih.gov/15250815/**

Alison Hayes, "Ableism in society: everybody wants you to be okay," Thriving While Disabled, April 9, 2021, **https://thrivingwhiledisabled.com/ableism-in-society-everybody-wants-you-to-be-okay/**.

Stress management

Alison Hayes, "Taking Care of Yourself During Stressful Times," Thriving While Disabled, August 3, 2018, **https://thrivingwhiledisabled.com/taking-care-of-yourself-during-stressful-times/**.

Alison Hayes, "Radical Self-care: Healing In Mind And Body," Thriving While Disabled, February 22, 2019, **https://thrivingwhiledisabled.com/radical-self-care/**.

RESOURCES WEBPAGE » CHAPTER 7

CHAPTER 8

Pacing

Pacing: The best way to budget your own reduced energy levels!

Let's get to something you can more directly control!

As I mentioned previously, when and as you become disabled or recognize you are managing a disabling condition, your energy levels are going to decrease in some way, shape, or form. You are going to need to create a "new normal" for yourself, because the old normal isn't going to work anymore. To summarize what most doctors tell patients early in their treatment: "You need to pace yourself."

Often, that's the entire statement and you're left wondering, "Okay, but what does that actually MEAN, and how am I supposed to do it?"

This is such an important topic and one too many of us gloss over because in some ways it's stupidly obvious, but in others, it's horribly opaque. Generally, pacing is the act of controlling your activities in such a way that you can manage them for a longer period of time, usually a pre-specified one.

Pace yourself to get through the whole test (meaning skip over a particularly difficult question to go back to if you have time, or make sure that you take enough time to read each question thoroughly), or pace yourself to get through the marathon (don't run so fast at the beginning you're too tired to finish the race, but not so slow you'll never catch up).

When there's a goal and a time limit, pacing is relatively self-explanatory. But pacing with a chronic condition or a long-term injury doesn't fully make sense, does it?

The goal of pacing is to be able to do more of the things, especially the things important to you and necessary for your quality of life, without becoming exhausted (physically, mentally, or emotionally) or unable to do anything more.

Recognize your triggers and their severity

Let's start with recognizing what triggers your symptoms, fatigues you, or otherwise makes it difficult for you to carry on.

In my case, for example, uncertainty and stress tend to trigger my FND symptoms. I have some very specific concepts/objects (like ladders and ambulances) that trigger my symptoms due to mental associations (both are strongly associated with my father's death).

The lower my overall stress level, and the less stress in my life, the better able I am to handle my specific triggers. Stress includes exercise, hunger, fatigue, extreme cold or heat, crowded spaces, excitement (yes, positive stress is a thing too) or feeling alone (depression trigger). It's all about balance for me and trying to stay within certain parameters to minimize my FND symptoms.

For my partner Al, his hip pain is generally triggered or worsened by holding certain positions (for example, driving becomes more painful over time due to him sitting and not changing position), so for him mitigation is about breaks, stretching, and changing up activities. Stooping, bending, and kneeling are more apt to be triggering. He is highly sensitive to cold and wet weather, so winter is more challenging for him than summer, and rainy days increase his pain level. Snowy days are very painful for him. We both know this and try to lower our expectations on those days.

For a blind person, triggers are likely to be activities they assume requires sight, but they can mitigate that by learning adaptive techniques to manage those challenges—so the more aware and comfortable they are with those adaptive tools, the fewer triggering events they will experience.

With something like food allergies or sensitivities, your time is best spent learning to recognize just what those sensitivities are, and where your triggering foods might hide. For you, pacing may be about focusing on what you are eating, with contingency plans to pace yourself around the extra energy you're putting into dietary planning and food prep, and the steps you need to take if your allergy is triggered.

Take some time to list the triggers you are aware of in your case and take note of anything you already do to mitigate those triggers. You may want to list possible triggers with ideas on how to test or measure them. The more aware you are of your triggers and their impact, the better you can plan for them.

Create your To-Do list and categorize your activities

Every day you wake up with a mental "to-do" list. The things you need or want to do, for yourself and for others.

You can divide the tasks you need to do into three different categories: recuperative/self-care (things that help you feel better), mental tasks (like making doctor's appointments, fighting insurance, figuring out finances, or writing), and physical tasks (like washing dishes, exercising, folding laundry, or participating in a sport).

Depending on the severity of your condition and where you are in your healing process, each of these will look very different. Early on, or with something especially severe, your recuperative/self-care activities may be lying in bed in the dark or taking a nap, but there will be points where your recuperative activities may be things like watching TV or reading or going for a walk in the woods.

The point is that your recuperative activities are what YOU need to feel better and be able to handle more, not what somebody else suggests you do (the exception being medical professionals who you know, like, and trust).

Depending on what you are managing, your mental and physical activities will adjust over time, as will what you expect of yourself. Early on (or during a flare or relapse) just getting out of bed may be a huge struggle, or you may struggle to maintain focus on any activity.

Later, those same actions may not require much (if any) thought or effort on your part, and you'll have different challenges to manage. The point of pacing is to recognize where you are RIGHT NOW and create a plan to rebuild at a pace you can handle and won't worsen your situation.

Look back at your list of triggers and recognize that many of those mitigating steps you wrote down are your recuperative activities.

Moving through your activities at the right pace

With pacing, your goal is to alternate through these three types of activities throughout the day, always stopping before you get fatigued or symptomatic.

For example, my recuperative activities include meditating, doing PT exercises, taking my medication on time, reading a book, watching TV, playing a video game, or walking in nature (when it's warm enough). If I'm especially fatigued, a nap may be in order.

My primary mental activity is my work related to **Thriving While Disabled** and this book, but I may need to make appointments for myself or Al, make plans with friends or family, or make insurance-related decisions or calls.

My main physical activities are exercising at the gym, going for walks, and handling household chores.

Generally, I could do mental activities for much of the day, but staying still for long periods isn't good for anybody's health, so I make a point of setting timers and doing other things in between rounds of mental activity.

So, I'll get up in the morning and meditate (sometimes it turns into a nap if I'm tired, but that's okay), have breakfast, and take my medications.

I spend much of the day (if I don't have outside commitments) working for 50-minute stretches with 10-minute "breaks" in between where I do household chores, PT exercises, or try to tidy up around the apartment.

If my focus or mental state slips, I usually shift into other regenerative activities to help pull myself out of the funk before it gets bad, and then after Al gets home from work, we go to the gym together several days a week.

I go to bed relatively early (climb into bed at 10 to read in hopes of falling asleep around 11 or so) in an attempt to re-establish a good sleep routine, since that is a challenge for me (as it is for many others with disabilities).

When I'm having bad symptom days, I can't do as much, so I try to get a bead on what I can do.

I may only work on things for shorter periods of time (maybe I can only work for half an hour at a time instead of an hour), or I try to simplify the routine (I may not go to the gym, but try to take a walk instead, or I may decrease the intensity or length of time I exercise).

If it's a really bad day symptom-wise, I may be lucky if I get anything beyond my recuperative activities done.

My goal through all of this is to be okay with whatever I can do (so no beating myself up for not getting everything done) and get myself back to my standard expectations as quickly and safely as possible.

When you're thinking about your situation, consider your current recuperative, physical, and mental activities. How can you balance them, and what are your priorities?

Rebuilding after the flare, shift, or diagnosis

For some disabled folks, there's a single setback and then their path to healing is relatively straightforward. I'm definitely not one of those people.

My FND is extremely stress-responsive and so every new trauma, crisis, or stress point in my life can severely increase my symptoms or lead to me developing new, sometimes completely different symptoms.

I've had a lot of practice of being held back and then trying to recover AGAIN. It does feel very frustrating.

Properly done, pacing helps reduce that stress, gives you a clearer path towards recovery, and reduces the likelihood and frequency of being stuck in a boom-and-bust cycle.

You know, where you feel good one day, so you do ALL THE THINGS (boom), then spend the next day/week/month being unable to do anything (bust)?

Breaking that habit helps you create a more predictable and manageable life.

I'm all for it, but pacing can be hard to do, especially because there are so many fun things out there that are made without disability in mind.

You can use pacing as a tool to help you slowly rebuild your stamina so you have a better sense of what you can and can't do safely, and to help you reduce how often you go boom-then-bust by planning ahead for fatiguing events/activities with extra recuperation time both before and after the event or activity.

For example, I've gone to weddings, conferences, holiday celebrations, and other activities knowing that they were more than I'd be able to handle on an ongoing basis.

However, I could rest up the day (or week) before and have low expectations for myself for a few days afterward and be able to thoroughly participate in that day or those days.

It's not ideal, but by pacing most of the time, you'll be able to recover from that cycle more quickly, and have it happen less often.

After getting Covid in 2022, I found myself not only having more FND symptoms than usual, but being a lot more emotionally volatile than usual. I'd jump from happy to depressed in moments, and was emotionally hypersensitive, especially to other people's emotions.

For me at that time, pacing wasn't just about balancing mental, physical, and recuperative tasks, but about controlling the emotions I was exposed to and creating emotional escapes for myself. I found even my tastes in TV shows to watch shifted because of the intensity of my emotional sensitivity.

Most of that has subsided now, but I'm still hesitant to risk exposure to the things that were most disruptive. When it came to physically managing my increase in FND symptoms, pacing was exactly what I needed.

At the gym, I reduced how long I was on the exercise bike in one stretch, and was able to get close to the same amount of time on the bike once I divided it into two periods of riding instead of one long one.

My PT helped me plan slowly increasing the length of the first period to retrain my brain to be okay with doing one long set again, by shifting things five minutes at a time.

I became stricter on stopping my work when the timer went off and doubled down on improving my sleep hygiene.

Expecting changes and managing your expectations

Is pacing going to make you able to do everything and anything?

Of course not. But it will help you be able to live a better-quality life than you would if you paced incorrectly or didn't bother trying to pace at all.

By investing some mental effort into planning your days and activities, you can get more done in the same amount of time with fewer symptoms and flares. By breaking up your activities into pieces your body and brain can handle, you prevent the fatigue or other triggers that have caused your symptom flares in the past. You can develop a better sense of what your limits are and what you can handle, and you can use pacing to slowly ramp up your activities so you have a more consistent idea of just what you can safely handle and what is too much of a push for you now.

You're more likely to be able to recognize and respect your limits, rather than constantly cycling between overdoing it and recovering from overdoing it. That combination is never going to lead to true recovery or a good sense of what you can and can't handle.

If instead you plan ahead and pace yourself, you can slowly and carefully discover your limits, have much smaller flares and much simpler corrections and spend most of your days feeling better than you otherwise would.

You absolutely can pace when dealing with mental health issues too. As I mentioned, my bout with Covid did a lot more damage to my mental health than my physical. I could feel my anxiety ratcheting up and my tolerance for certain types of stress dropping dramatically.

I took time to recognize what was happening and to notice my new mental health triggers. I discussed it with my psychiatrist and adjusted my medications slightly.

I shifted the type of meditation I was doing, from exercises on controlling my body to more exercises focused on my mindset and processing my emotions. I took time to examine my feelings, what triggered them, and how I could manage them. I got support in this from my therapist as well.

Just like in managing my physical health, I recognized my triggers and avoided them until I could recuperate and explore other management methods.

In the meantime, I continued to alternate through recuperative, mental, and physical activities, but with a recognition that my thought process and emotions were a bit unreliable, so I was prepared to shift things as needed, and potentially place more emphasis on my recuperative activities than I normally would.

Anxiety or depression can easily sneak up on you when dealing with the unknown, and the world of chronic illness is full of unknowns and uncertainties. If, like me, you've spent much of your life managing a mental illness, you know that state of mind has a huge impact on what you are able to get yourself to do, and how many spoons (we'll discuss spoons in the next major section) you have available for getting things done.

Pacing your way through this series

These books are full of mental activities that you will need to take to survive and then thrive while managing your condition/s. You are constantly going to be balancing your needs, determining how much of your precious energy you can afford to spend on each program you might apply for, and compare that to the cost of not having that support. I know this. I support you in that journey. You can and will create the patterns that help you succeed in these processes without causing yourself further harm.

As I mentioned in the foreword, I highly recommend taking the time to glance through the table of contents for this book (and Volume II when you read it) and to dip into whatever sections you need at any given point in time! This volume is full of information that may shift how you view the world and may require multiple read-throughs to absorb. The second volume is full of programs, laws, and rules that may protect you or help you survive, but they will take energy to understand or apply for, and due to structural ableism, may well take more effort and energy than they first appear to.

I hope that my suggestions and information help you prioritize what needs to be done to give you the best chance of success and to manage your expectations for any program or law you use or depend on.

I know how much I would have been helped by being introduced to a deeper understanding of pacing earlier in my own disability acceptance process and want to be sure you have access as soon as possible so you can apply it to your life!

KEY POINTS

- **Pacing** is the process of working within your limits so that you can do more activities with fewer costs. It is highly personalized and based on your current limitations.

CHAPTER 9

Disability Culture and Tropes

Disability Culture

As I mentioned in Chapter 2, disability history and culture are hard to grasp and even more difficult to pass on to the next generation, but I do want to talk about the ideas and more universal concepts and beliefs many members of the disability community are aware of, share, or use.

We don't usually gather physically, many of us are both geographically and/or socially isolated, and we often are siloed away from one another because so much of disability is medicalized (so we gather based on diagnosis or symptoms). I hope work will continue to help unite the entire disability community, rather than just subsections of it.

This volume is not a definitive guide to disability culture, but it is the gathering of information and experiences that I personally am aware of. I would love to learn and share more! As my book does have a website-based component, I would love to hear from you if you know of more resources I should be aware of, or other disability thought leaders I should learn about! I'll be mentioning people throughout the books, but know my list is far from complete.

There are some useful disability-related terms that you should know. And I'm not talking about names of diseases or medications or treatment plans. I'm talking about descriptions of coping techniques, dangerous thought processes, and biases that frequently impact our community!

So, let's start with the common beliefs about people with disabilities so that you can immediately counter them when they forcibly collide with you, then close out with some words and concepts to add to your vocabulary so you can join in on discussions that use disability shorthand!

Disability mythology

These are the biases and misunderstandings that underlie a lot of ableist thoughts and actions. My aim throughout this section is to point out the stories society tells us, so we can remind ourselves they simply are not true.

1. **Disability is an excuse or failure**

    This is a pretty pervasive story, stuck in our collective unconscious. Too many people interpret the term "disability" itself in this light. "Dis" as a prefix is generally viewed as a negative term, and "ability" is viewed as such a positive one (think about it, how often has the term "ability" been used negatively in your life? "Skill" and "ability" are almost universally expressed as positive things to have or collect), that even the concept of disability feels taboo, with too many people trying to avoid its use.

    Ableism is deeply entrenched in our society, and it's much easier, emotionally, for abled people to say that disabilities aren't real than it is to recognize they, too could become disabled themselves. If somebody who was a hard worker, or very expressive, or mentally sharp, suddenly now isn't, then that's something that could happen to anyone, including the abled person noticing the change in their colleague or loved one.

    The idea that that difference cannot be fixed is even worse, so it's much easier for abled people who aren't deeply involved to assume disabled people in general are scapegoating or not trying hard enough, rather than to recognize that no, we really can't do the thing anymore (or doing the thing isn't worth the cost), which means that they might reach a point when they can't either. This is effectively recognizing one's own mortality, and people simply don't want to do that. So, in too many cases, they simply don't.

2. **Disabled people are child-like**

   This is another negative stereotype of disabled people that causes all kinds of damage to relationships between disabled and abled people, or between disabled people with different disabilities.

   After all, just because we unlearn crap about our own conditions, doesn't mean we understand the mindset or needs of people with completely different conditions, especially with how divided our community tends to be.

   This idea comes out in a huge variety of ways and causes all kinds of damage. Examples of various forms of this bias include disabled people aren't sexual beings, disabled people can't/shouldn't have children, disabled people are their family's responsibility, disabled people can't live independently, disabled people are unemployable, or disabled people are burdens—plus many other variations. Basically, the idea underlying a lot of bias against people with disabilities, is this tendency to equate us with children.

   Now, certain disabilities can leave some of us with some behaviors, capacities, or traits similar to children, but the comparison is inaccurate and hurtful. The images and ideas around us being child-like are socially damaging and disempowering.

   Consider the many disabled people looking to date and/or have sex, disabled people in emotionally unsafe or unhealthy families, parents with disabilities, and so on who need to put extra effort into breaking down these stereotypes on top of all the other considerations they are dealing with. Recognize this stereotype whenever you see or experience it, so you can avoid applying it to others, and call out people who are making this ableist assumption.

3. **Disability is contagious**

   There are many contagious diseases out there. However, most disabling conditions are not associated with contagious conditions, and many that are don't necessarily mean that the person with the condition is likely to infect another person. The few long-term diseases that remain contagious generally are harder to share than people assume.

   People tend to strongly associate disability with illness, and this is one of the side effects of that association.

   This is more likely to happen with people who operate with minimal information or education, but even in areas with higher levels of education and information sharing, you still see the occasional person recoil from or avoid a person with a disability because of this bias.

4. **People with disabilities are fragile or weak**

   This is somewhat related to the childlike imagery, but I did want to mention it separately. Many of the older synonyms for at least some disabilities are very direct in drawing this line. For example, pregnant women used to be referred to as being in "delicate condition" during Victorian times, many people with chronic illnesses have historically been described as having "weak constitutions" or generally being frail.

   While some of us might tire more quickly, have our bodies (or mobility equipment) break or fail to work more often, or may be slower to process or respond to information, we often are similar to our abled peers in most other ways.

   It requires emotional resilience and other forms of strength to keep living and fighting when even our own bodies and/or minds seem to turn against us. I understand that abled people often see or presume that we are weak, but they often miss the many types of strengths we have!

5. **People with disabilities are disabled as a lesson or curse and/or people who are disabled deserve it!**

   Think back to the moral model of disability we discussed in Chapter 2! This happens too often, especially with religious groups.

   Having a disability is sometimes framed as the result of damage to a person's soul, a test of their spiritual strength, or a curse due to someone's (usually the mother's) poor choices or sinful behavior. The disability is painted as either a punishment (to the disabled individual or their family) or a test (of the disabled individual or their family). In some way or other, their disability happened for a reason and so the disabled individual (and/or their family) are not worthy of community support.

   This allows members of the community to avoid or minimize any sense of guilt or responsibility they would otherwise feel.

   A variation on this theme is people feeling the need to publicly pray for disabled individuals, in hopes their deity will heal or forgive that person.

   There are occasionally disabled people who believe their God gave them their disability as a test or lesson, and sometimes will claim they were healed after learning that lesson.

A few symbols related to disability

Sunflowers (invisible disabilities): The sunflower as representation for invisible illnesses started in the UK a few years ago, and has been adopted in various ways to various degrees throughout Europe and beyond. This was started in 2016 and has been slowly expanding.

> 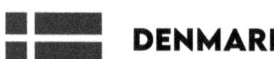 **DENMARK**
>
> In Denmark, a friend shared that the sunflower has been used to denote easy access for people with invisible conditions, with some stores having checkout lines specifically for people with a sunflower lanyard or pin (a free lanyard is available for people self-identifying as invisibly disabled).

Wheelchair user (blue background white wheelchair symbol): The official symbol for disabled/accessible zones for people with disabilities.

Puzzle pieces have been used to represent the Autism spectrum(and sometimes other disabilities), but too often that has been viewed as ableist as it's associated with presuming people on the autism spectrum are incomplete or broken, when ASD is better thought of as an expansion of the range of human experience. Some organizations that use the puzzle piece symbology are seeking a cure or follow other practices currently viewed as ableist. Approach the puzzle piece symbology with caution as the group may be well-intentioned but may hold ableist perspectives on the disabilities they support. I'm not saying all will, just to do your due diligence if this symbol is being used. A **sideways rainbow infinity symbol** is often used by the Autistic community, and is more acceptable.

Disability-based Culture

There can be culture around specific disabilities. The Deaf community is the easiest example of this. Notice I capitalized Deaf and through the books I will tend to capitalize the word or do things like d/Deaf. This is because Deaf culture is a very real thing. I am not part of Deaf culture and do not have personal experience with it, but I want people to be aware there is a sense of community among people with similar or overlapping disabilities, and some of those are strong enough to become a unique culture.

What I do know of Deaf culture is that they tend to be very upfront and free of BS. Deaf culture includes language (ASL in the US), behavior, and cultural norms, as well as community values and expectations.

The Deaf community can hold itself somewhat separate from the larger disability community as some Deaf people do not consider themselves disabled. Hearing people born into families where one or more parents are Deaf sometimes choose to identify as culturally Deaf due to their participation in the Deaf community.

There is something unique and special about this identity and community that I want us all to recognize, something I suspect is partly because deafness can be inherited and passed down, combined with the historical tendency to send deaf children off to be educated primarily with other deaf children. Schools specifically for deaf children have been around at least since the early 1800s, likely longer, so there has been time and space for Deaf culture to grow.

For the rest of us disabled people, there often are identity groups, support groups, or other opportunities to create a community based on commonality of needs (wheelchair users, for example) or diagnosis (I've had periods of being active within the FND community). We all deserve community and have multiple ways to create or participate in it.

Many resources are most likely to be found online, as that tends to be the easiest way to connect and the method that is least likely to be tiring. This means disability-based groups often end up becoming international simply as a result of being similarly accessible to people around the world. We all deserve community and support, so please look for other disabled groups based on your own needs, diagnosis/es, or identity!

Let's recognize Inspiration Porn

This term was coined by Stella Young in her TedTalk "I'm not your inspiration" (the link is in the resources section). Inspiration porn includes images, stories, or news bites about people with disabilities doing ordinary things.

These often feature an abled "hero" helping a disabled "victim", aiming to help the (abled) audience feel better about themselves, and rarely actually helping the disability community. Examples of inspiration porn include those stories about high school or college students creating a wheelchair for a young child whose parents couldn't afford to buy them one (rather than focusing on the insurance company's refusal to cover the chair), stories of an abled person (often a white, young woman) either asking a disabled person (usually a young man with a severe developmental, intellectual, or information processing disability) to go to prom with her, or (sometimes a mom) creating a special version of a school social event for one or more disabled people.

Basically, inspiration porn is focused on either celebrating a non-achievement by a disabled person (such as an expected graduation or other life milestone) or an abled person's "normalizing" of a disabled person's participation in such a milestone (usually by creating an alternative version). Almost all news stories about or related to disabled individuals follow the inspiration porn trope to some degree, using the disabled individual/s primarily as props for the story of the abled person or group who helped them.

Another common theme in news related to disabled people are stories painting us as the victims of mistreatment or abuse, which is scarcely better.

Recognizing the Supercrip

Supercrips are disabled people who go above and beyond all reasonable expectations. Supercrips have degrees and partners and money and run multiple businesses, or are amazing athletes, or otherwise are more successful than most abled people, let alone other minorities and/or disabled people.

A supercrip is an individual who has achieved much more than most abled people do, usually because they are that level of driven, or because they are fictional. The supercrip can be related to inspiration porn, as supercrips are often held up as amazing success stories, used to shame average abled people, essentially saying, "This person is so successful despite their disability...what's your excuse?"

Supercrips are not bad people in and of themselves (the ones who exist tend to be extremely motivated people who have made some form of sacrifice and/or grew up in positions of relative privilege), but their stories are too often used to inspire abled people to try harder and increase the feelings of failure in average, everyday disabled folks.

Being in the public eye, supercrips, like most famous people, have the ability to curate their story so outsiders don't necessarily see the struggles they face/d.

Supercrips parallel abled ultimate success stories—the person who succeeded may not be a bad or ill-intentioned person, but too many people wield these success stories as an unrealistic model for others to follow. Yes, they **succeed** despite the odds, but they succeeded **despite the odds**, so there's no sense expecting every person who shares their diagnosis or symptoms to be as successful, just like it's not reasonable to expect such an extreme level of success from all members of any other identity group.

Beware of Toxic Positivity

Toxic positivity is what occurs when healthy optimism, gratitude, and positive thinking concepts are taken to an unhealthy extreme. Disabled people are not the only people to experience toxic positivity (usually from abled people), but we are one of the minorities most likely to experience it, and we often experience it on multiple fronts.

Toxic positivity appears in statements like "good vibes only" or encouragement to smile or put on a happy face no matter what is happening. We experience toxic positivity when consistently told to look on the bright side, or that "others have it worse" when we mention struggles we are facing. Toxic positivity occurs when realistic assessments and valid emotional responses are painted as unhealthy or overly pessimistic. Toxic positivity includes minimizing a person's emotional experience.

All emotions can be healthy and so-called negative emotions can be appropriate responses to difficult situations. While getting trapped or stuck in difficult emotions isn't healthy, it's similarly unhealthy to ignore your emotional response to difficult events. Toxic positivity can be a response anyone receives to sharing emotional responses viewed as "negative", but as people with disabilities frequently have to share difficult health news and can rarely honestly state their health is good (which can negatively impact our mental health), we are extra likely to be repeatedly targeted by multiple people for variations of toxic positivity.

As disabled people, we are dealing with being minimized. Toxic positivity when directed at us is a form of societal gaslighting and should be treated that way.

Spoon Theory

I want to briefly mention another concept I refer to at points in the book, which is "spoon theory". You may have seen people with disabilities (especially energy or mental health associated ones) referring to themselves as spoonies or mentioning having (or more frequently running out of) spoons. Christine Miserandino coined the concept, and it's been eagerly adopted and adapted.

On the most basic level, spoons are simply units of energy, the combination of physical ability and mental capacity to do something. A person who is out of spoons doesn't have the energy to do anything (picture sprawling on a couch, exhausted, unable to even turn on the TV, read a book, or use their smartphone). Many things that abled people take for granted or only consider in terms of time (like taking a shower, eating, or brushing their teeth) can take up much more energy when you are managing a disability.

Disabilities often lead people to start their days with less energy with which to do these things, and more uncertainty about how much energy they will have on any given day. All of these factors together means that people with disabilities become much more likely to run out of energy and/or will power before the end of the day.

Spoons are a shorthand for that combination of energy and will-power abled folks take for granted because the exhaustion of running out of spoons happens much less frequently (if at all). Examples of times when abled people might have a similar experience will be extreme loss (like losing a child) or severe illness or injury (AKA being temporarily disabled).

Many disabled people, in contrast, regularly run low on spoons or need to focus and think about their priorities so they don't run out of spoons on a regular (sometimes daily) basis. Also, for disabled people, concerns over spoons are a life-long experience, rather than a temporary situation.

I have a link in the resources section to the original blog post on spoon theory, and to the initial blog post on fork theory, which I discuss next.

Fork Theory

Fork theory was created by Jen Rose, a member of the neurodiversity community, to describe the irritations and distractions (and worse) in life that will eventually lead to a meltdown, as well as the idea that one solution for the associated overwhelm is to remove the more manageable discomforts so you can process other issues.

Think about the phrase "stick a fork in me, I'm done" and visualize all different sizes of forks, from the tiny escargot fork of a hangnail to a pitchfork like your best friend saying the most hurtful thing possible at the worst possible moment.

You may be able to handle many small forks, but zero large ones. As members of the disability community, we may be dealing with more forks more often, but everybody experiences these stresses.

Our experiences of ableism are a collection of forks just waiting to poke us, and we run a high risk of running out of spoons to handle these stresses.

I'm afraid that any social welfare or disability-related program you may apply for will provide way too many forks and use up more spoons than you'd like, but I'm telling you about them since you may well need them to get yourself to a better, more stable life.

The most important thing to remember throughout the process is that most (if not all) of the frustration and confusion you will be facing is not due to some inherent weakness or failure on your part, but rather is the result of societal ableism, classism, and bureaucratic incompetence.

KEY POINTS

- **Disabled people** as a group are not childlike, weak, failures, or morally inferior to abled people.

- **Inspiration porn** occurs when a disabled person is either celebrated for doing totally normal things or used as a prop to celebrate an abled person's willingness to help them.

- **Supercrips** are people with disabilities who have succeeded in life in some remarkable way and whose stories are often misused to shame or "encourage" others.

- **Toxic positivity:** The insistence on always maintaining a positive mindset/discouraging "negative" emotions even in the face of reality.

- **Spoons** refer to units of mental and emotional energy, particularly relevant to the disability community.

- **Forks** represent irritants and challenges that can lead to emotional breakdowns. Removing them reduces stress. Introduced by a member of the neurodiverse community.

RESOURCES

Admin, "Deaf Culture 101: Traditions, Values & Communication," Deaf Websites, 2023, **https://deafwebsites.com/deaf-culture-101-traditions-values-communication/**.

Claire Stanley, "What I Want You to Understand About the 'Supercrip' Stereotype," The Mighty, published December 22, 2015, last updated March 4, 2024, **https://themighty.com/topic/blindness/challenging-the-supercrip-stereotype-of-people-with-disabilities/**.

Alison Hayes, "Toxic Positivity Vs Realistic Optimism: Knowing The Difference!," Thriving While Disabled, September 13, 2019, **https://thrivingwhiledisabled.com/toxic-positivity-vs-realistic-optimism-knowing-the-difference/**.

Christine Miserandino, "The Spoon Theory," But You Don't Look Sick, copyright 2025, **https://butyoudontlooksick.com/articles/written-by-christine/the-spoon-theory/**.

Jen Rose, "Fork Theory," Jen Rose, December 15, 2018, **https://jenrose.com/fork-theory/**.

RESOURCES WEBPAGE » CHAPTER 9

CHAPTER 10

Practicing Mindful Self-Compassion

Practicing Mindful Self-Compassion

What can you do in response to all the stresses society is adding to your already full plate? You may benefit from exploring mindfulness and mindful self-compassion. Mindfulness is the ability to live in the moment—not thinking about the future or the past but simply being aware of the sensations and activities you are experiencing right now.

Mindful self-compassion is the practice of being self-aware in the moment and practicing kindness and empathy to yourself while you are there.

I have always been a somewhat anxious person who thinks ahead to problem solve, and I have had periods where I was very focused on traumatic and stressful events that had happened to me. By doing that, I compounded a lot of my pain.

I have done a lot of work on picking apart different events in my life, and being able to separately acknowledge the losses, instead of being in an emotional tangle of hurt and sadness. I have learned to let myself grieve and then get back into the flow of life.

I definitely did not have those skills as a child and young adult. I now spend less of my time and emotional energy on my past and things that went wrong, and more of it on focusing on my present life.

How does mindful meditation help?

Meditation and mindfulness are evidence-based rational routines that can help you focus more on yourself and your body and your emotions, allowing you to increase your self-awareness and better know who you really are. When you are more self-aware, you can build or rebuild your life in directions that can make you truly happy.

If you do not work on your self-awareness and figuring out your own bodily needs, it's easy to fall into the trap of escapism. I have watched people lose themselves in TV shows (or any other obsession) and know others do it through drug abuse. They don't improve, they don't try to make themselves better, and they stay stuck, unable to truly heal.

There is a specific program, Mindfulness-Based Stress Reduction (MBSR), which was originally created in 1979 by Jon Kabat-Zinn to help patients with chronic pain to better manage their symptoms and improve their quality of life. It has since been found to be incredibly useful for people with a wide range of physical, mental, and emotional challenges and differences. One of my neurologists had recommended that I explore it to help me manage my FND symptoms. It has been quite helpful, and the resources section includes a link to a free MBSR course that I found online and participated in.

MBSR and mindfulness practices have proven to be very helpful tools for many people (both abled and disabled), helping you to better understand yourself, manage physical and/or emotional pain, and learn to relax and slow down, a skill that has become much more difficult for society in the past 50 years or so than it was in the more distant past.

Is mindfulness THE solution? Of course not, but it can be a useful tool. And, like most powerful treatments, mindfulness can have unexpected side effects. While most people who practice mindfulness find it helpful and healing, there are a percentage of people who may develop new mental health issues or simply not experience much improvement[36.] I

---

36 Jarrett, Dan. "Meditation and Mindfulness Have a Dark Side That We Don't Talk About." ScienceAlert. Published November 11, 2021. Accessed April 10, 2025. **https://www.sciencealert.com/meditation-and-mindfulness-have-a-dark-side-that-we-dont-talk-about**.

am mentioning the risk here since many individuals and organizations that discuss mindfulness practices may deny the possibility of a negative reaction to the exercise. For most people, the practice of mindfulness is helpful, healing, and informative, but if you find the practice of mindfulness to truly trigger an unhealthy reaction (as opposed to the discomfort that may accompany processing or recognizing your reactions or identity), that is absolutely a valid reason to stop practice and explore other treatment options.

Self-compassion

Self-compassion is another vital healing process. It's something only you can do for yourself, and as such, it is a predominantly internal process.

When you think about your actions, processes, health, and life, how critical are you? How quickly? Self-compassion is the ability to be kind to yourself and caring, just like you would be to a friend.

I have a long history of being afraid of being abandoned and therefore not wanting to be alone. When I found myself home alone, I would often start feeling anxious or feel like I couldn't enjoy anything I tried to do—the feeling of loneliness (and of being unloved and unlovable) would kick in and I would get angry with myself for making it worse. That, of course, would reinforce the fear of being alone and the feeling of being unlovable, so the issue would compound itself rapidly.

If instead, I had been able to connect more with my self-compassion, I could have been able to soothe myself with better thoughts—I was only alone for a few hours, my partner/family/friends still loved me, I was safe and deserved to enjoy myself. The better I could feel at that moment, the easier it would be for me to shake off those fears and anxieties. The negative self-talk I did to myself was the main thing increasing my stress and agitation.

The more self-compassionate I could be, the easier that time alone was. By being compassionate to myself, I am better able to enjoy what I am doing and able to recover much more gracefully from situations I don't like.

Self-compassion is one of those skills too many of us (abled people included) are low on, and internalized ableism tends to reduce our self-compassion even further. Taking the time to recognize both our likelihood to be overly judgmental of ourselves and our increased need for self-compassion can help us along on our healing journeys.

Why am I talking about mindful self-compassion here?

When living with a disability, there are a lot of additional stresses on us. Financially, we often have reduced income and increased medical expenses after the onset or increase in the severity of our conditions. Physically, many of us have an increase in physical pain or limitations due to our conditions. If we are dealing with a mental health issue, our thought process is affecting our ability to live day by day. If the disability isn't directly mental health-related, the acceptance of the physical issues we are managing is apt to trigger some mental health challenges. Socially, our conditions often affect our relationship with those around us.

Becoming disabled (and accepting our disability/ies) is a huge adjustment, and the mental and emotional toll of managing all that stress often slows our healing process or makes it more challenging.

The ableism that exists in modern society compounds all these issues. Self-compassion is essential for us as we are going through the process of accepting our conditions and improving our coping skills. We now have this (additional) minority identity, adding to the stress and discrimination we are likely to face daily.

Mindfulness, especially Mindfulness-Based Stress Reduction (MBSR), can be a powerful tool in our own healing processes and help us mentally readjust to our disabled identities. Self-compassion is always important and useful for emotional healing, and societal messaging reinforces the idea that we, as disabled people, are even less deserving of self-compassion than we were when we were (or identified as) abled.

As mentioned earlier, pacing is an important skill to help you better manage your life. Practicing mindfulness will help you better listen to your body and be more aware of what is "too much" for you in the moment, so you can minimize your symptoms/flares. Practicing self–compassion will help you reduce the stress you experience, help you recognize and counter your internalized ableism more quickly, and give you a better chance of noticing the positives in your life.

Living with mindful self-compassion

Through mindfulness, we can better recognize our physical and emotional needs, become more self-aware, and in many cases be better able to articulate our needs and desires. Once we learn these things about ourselves, practicing self-compassion helps us to handle these in a constructive way, and helps our healing, rather than seeing failure and berating ourselves for it.

By recognizing myself, my limits, and my needs using mindfulness, I am quicker to realize when I'm out of sync with myself or when I'm not doing well, which can often help me self-correct without a physical or emotional crash (or with a much smaller one).

By practicing self-compassion, I'm more resilient each time something stressful occurs. I am managing the problem, as opposed to solving the problem while beating myself up emotionally, then needing to figure out how to put myself back together after that.

If you have rarely experienced compassion from others the situation is even more challenging, but that means it's a skill worth developing in yourself. If you focus on this, you can be better in touch with yourself and your feelings, heal better and more completely, and are much more likely to be able to enjoy your life.

Applying mindful self-compassion to your life

Meditation and mindfulness are both very good techniques to care for yourself. The idea of being still and focusing inward is very important because many of us are very distanced from our bodies and our needs. There are so many things outside of ourselves vying for our attention that we need to actively set aside time to just "be", and mindful self-compassion is a way to "be" while being more self-aware, being able to connect with your own needs and desires, and unknotting the tangle your emotions are in.

We have had more than enough experiences to make us more self-critical. We (as a society) are too used to escapism instead of facing our problems. By understanding ourselves, we have the best possible chance to really enjoy our lives. So, when you feel stressed or frightened by your situation:

Let it go.

Breathe.

Just focus on being you and knowing who you are and what you want. The better you know yourself, the better you know your needs and desires, the easier it is for you to determine what your next right step in life is, and the happier you are likely to be.

And doesn't everybody, deep down, just want to be happy?

KEY POINTS

- **Mindfulness** includes being focused on everything as it happens in the moment, rather than thinking about the future or the past.
- **Self-compassion** is the ability to kind to yourself the same way you would be to a friend. People tend to be much more critical of themselves than they are of people they care about.

RESOURCES

Mindful Self-Compassion Resources

"What Is Mindfulness?" Mindful.org. Accessed April 10, 2025. **https://www.mindful.org/what-is-mindfulness/**.

Palouse Mindfulness Free Online Course. Accessed April 10, 2025. **https://palousemindfulness.com/**.

Center for Mindful Self-Compassion. Accessed April 10, 2025. **https://centerformsc.org/**.

Hayes, Alison "Disability and Sleep Disorders." Thriving While Disabled. Accessed April 10, 2025. **https://thrivingwhiledisabled.com/disability-and-sleep-disorders/**.

Hayes, Alison "Gratitude Is the Best Attitude to Help You Heal." Thriving While Disabled. Accessed April 10, 2025. **https://thrivingwhiledisabled.com/gratitude-is-the-best-attitude-to-help-you-heal/**.

RESOURCES WEBPAGE » CHAPTER 10

SECTION 2

Disability Life Milestones

CHAPTER 11

Our Right as a Minority to Exist
Disabled lives are too often viewed as disposable

Historical (and sometimes modern) control over disabled people's lives and bodies

I need to start this conversation with the elephant in the room: people in power have historically policed disabled minds and bodies. The most obvious example was people with disabilities were the first identity group murdered by Nazis during World War II.[37] Institutionalized disabled people were the first group both passively (neglect) then actively (gas chambers) killed, and the program used for these murders was the model used for the later murders of other, by Nazi standards, "undesirables". The term used to describe the program? **Euthanasia.**

While this was one of the most concerted efforts to remove the disabled population from a country, it is far from the only time disabled people were targeted for removal from the gene pool.

Disabled people who are unable to live independently have tended to be institutionalized, which is where most of the worst offenses have tended to occur. The Nazi euthanasia programs started in these

---

37 "The Murder of People with Disabilities." United States Holocaust Memorial Museum Encyclopedia. Accessed April 10, 2025. **https://encyclopedia.ushmm.org/content/en/article/the-murder-of-people-with-disabilities**.

institutions, as have many other abuses on the disabled population. The Olmstead Decision of 1999[38] was the first law that enshrined the right of disabled people who need government support to survive to control where they live (i.e., to choose to live in the larger community rather than within an institution for people with disabilities).

There is a long history of reducing the reproductive freedom of people with disabilities (and people identified as being disabled). Besides the social costs attached to being disabled, many countries[39], including the US[40], have instituted sterilization programs for people with disabilities (and other undesirable populations).

This is not solely something that has happened in the past, it is an ongoing issue globally (yes, including within the US). These legally obtained, forced sterilizations are often built on a history of eugenics, ableism, and sometimes racism. In a percentage of the cases, the (predominantly) girls and women sterilized aren't aware of what has happened, and may have a legal guardian, which may prevent them from exercising other rights like voting, marrying, or controlling their medical care.

This is deeply entwined with sexism, because usually the population controlled this way are the people who get pregnant and give birth.

With this history in mind, I want to help you recognize the additional challenges I know the disability community faces when thinking about the right to die, abortion regulation, and the related topic of IVF treatment.

---

38 "About Olmstead." Olmstead Rights. Accessed April 10, 2025. **https://www.olmsteadrights.org/about-olmstead/**.
39 Neuhof, Anna. "Sterilization of Women and Girls with Disabilities." Human Rights Watch. News, November 10, 2011. Accessed April 10, 2025. **https://www.hrw.org/news/2011/11/10/sterilization-women-and-girls-disabilities**.
40 "Forced Sterilization of Disabled People in the United States." National Women's Law Center. Accessed April 10, 2025. **https://nwlc.org/resource/forced-sterilization-of-disabled-people-in-the-united-states/**.

Euthanasia and the right to die

While the United States of America currently does not allow euthanasia, it is a subject that comes up for debate from time to time. Dr. Kevorkian[41] was one of the more famous doctors who supported patients in this process, but there have always been people who may help people in this manner, and people who have taken such responsibilities into their own hands and "helped" people to die who may or may not have wanted it. (There's even a term for people who commit these sorts of murders, "angel of mercy" killers[42].)

What does this have to do with disability, you may ask. Well, generally, disability is the reason people consider and/or are "granted" death. They have been diagnosed with a condition that should (or will) end in death, and they believe the intervening time will be painful and worthless (or not worth the pain), so why not avoid the worst of the pain and end their life now?

In all honesty, I don't have a strong moral stance on an individual making this choice if it truly is their choice and there is no chance for recovery. My concern is that structural ableism is interfering in this process in a way that pushes people towards this decision, and the option of death is much easier to access than the help or support to understand and live with their condition.

---

41 Editors, Biography.com. "Jack Kevorkian." Biography.com. Updated April 9, 2021. Accessed April 10, 2025. **https://www.biography.com/scientists/jack-kevorkian**.
42 Parry, Owen. "Healthcare's Medical Serial Killers." Crime Traveller, June 2018. Accessed April 10, 2025. **https://www.crimetraveller.org/2018/06/healthcare-medical-serial-killers/**.

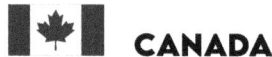 **CANADA**

MAiD (Medical Assistance in Dying) was passed in Canada, and it shows many of the problems that come with legalizing medically assisted suicide. Let's explore them now:

1. **Doctors are central to the process (conflict of interest and ableist biases).**

    Doctors are people. They are part of larger society and so frequently carry (and sometimes fail to recognize) the biases others have. This means they, too, often carry ableist beliefs, such as the idea that disabled lives are inherently less worthy, or that disabled people by definition have low quality of life. These biases serve to lower their assessment of the patient's quality of life or worthiness to live, and increase the risk the doctor will say or do things to discourage or fail to encourage their patient from continuing to fight for their survival.

    These factors highlight the fact that doctors are supposed to be the people most invested in helping their patients to survive and recover, and whose expertise is supposed to be in that survival and recovery. If/when euthanasia is legalized, what is there to prevent doctors from offering this as a solution for any patient who is grieving their diagnosis or who the doctor believes does not deserve to live (such as multiply-marginalized identities)?

    This puts additional emotional weight on doctors who may need to simultaneously advise their patient on treatment options and discuss the option of ending their lives. This issue becomes more apparent when we're discussing the intersection of these issues and considering doctors who already recommend inappropriate treatments to patients[43] without due thought or who are so opposed to admitting they don't have an answer that they create one.

---

43 Elliott, Brianna. "Almost 40% of women were not offered alternative treatments prior to a hysterectomy." Medical News Today. Published December 15, 2015. Accessed April 10, 2025. **https://www.medicalnewstoday.com/articles/287736**.

Given how biased the medical system currently is, adding the option of death to the available menu feels very ill-advised, at least until the challenges mentioned are resolved.

2. **Doctors have a great deal of power over their patients and too many people tend to put doctors on a pedestal and view them as more knowledgeable and less biased than they truly are.**

   Many people embrace doctor's statements of options as declarations of necessity and have inappropriate or unnecessary treatments based on one doctor's opinions. For example, the number of young women who get hysterectomies and therefore lose their fertility when it wasn't the appropriate treatment is staggering[44]. How can we guarantee that patients won't get similarly bad advice from their doctors when it comes to the even more permanent solution of euthanasia? Because it definitely will end the pain.

3. **Misdiagnoses happen, and new treatments and cures are being created every day.**

   Patients with tough diagnoses need time and education to truly understand what they are living with, and time to experiment with treatments, and understand the changes happening in their bodies. Time for treatments to be improved or new treatments to be developed is greatly reduced (as are opportunities to test the efficacy) if patients are immediately offered the option of dying instead. MAiD does take some steps to defend against this, but if it's easier to access doctors who provide this assistance than it is to see providers with the appropriate expertise in your condition, we have a problem.

---

44 Reinstein, Julie. "Are Doctors Performing Too Many Hysterectomies in America?" Shape. Published November 13, 2023. Accessed April 10, 2025. **https://www.shape.com/lifestyle/mind-and-body/overperforming-hysterectomy-in-america**.

4. **It is much easier (and cheaper) to access MAiD than any of the disability/survival assistance programs.**

    This effectively reinforces the argument that disabled lives are low value and deserve minimal consideration. Effectively, people with disabilities in Canada are being told if they want to live, they will need to get on lists, wait for months to years, and then maybe they'll get a percentage of the help they need. Or they can take the other path and be out of the picture rather quickly, so nobody needs to think about them again. It's a pretty ableist message and reinforces all the ableist messaging we've been discussing in this book. It reinforces capitalist messaging that to have value you must be employed/working, and if you lose that, you lose all value to society.

5. **Societal ableism means that people recently diagnosed often believe that death is the better option.**

    For the many reasons we discussed before, people newly diagnosed with permanently disabling conditions are grieving this major change in their lives and struggling with the ramifications of this change. They are low on spoons and overwhelmed. They may have espoused one of the ableist storylines many disabled people are exposed to: "If I were you/had your condition, I'd kill myself because your life isn't worth living." Well, during that period following symptoms and/or diagnosis, they may be much more likely to act on that belief, when they might not do so after some time to adjust to their new identity. It is good that they have a 90-day waiting period for people whose diagnoses are not imminently painfully fatal, but if that waiting period is similar in length to (or, worse, shorter than) the wait for social supports necessary for survival, it doesn't send the best message.

6. **Social support networks frequently fray or break during health crises, leaving individuals more likely to be alone/lonely, which can trigger suicidality or feelings of abandonment/worthlessness.**

   Reinforcing the previous point, many people experience social isolation and the loss of relationships they valued during this transitional time (as we discussed in Chapter 6), and those types of losses often lead them to consider death or otherwise escaping the pain of living. While there are security measures in place, I think the pain of societal ableism can be more debilitating than the condition itself. This is not to diminish the very real pain and frustration that accompanies many disabilities, especially more severe and painful ones.

7. **Ableism is so severe that too often people cheer on the idea of choosing to die, which puts increased social pressure on individuals to make this decision or carry through with the option if presented with it.**

   Along similar lines, many people with minority identities already have higher rates of suicide, mental illness, poor health outcomes, and/or trauma in their lives, and there are multiple organizations that work to reduce suicidality in these groups. Similar efforts should be made for people living with disabilities, rather than actively encouraging us to consider death as a treatment option.

8. **Many people living with chronic pain are fighting on a regular basis for appropriate treatments for their condition and are frequently treated with suspicion due to the opioid epidemic.**

   This again complicates matters as both pain and pain medicine can lower quality of life, impair decision-making ability, and impact the fight to be treated appropriately by medical professionals Again, the fatigue from the fight may become too much and increase the likelihood of finding death a viable alternative to the fight for support to manage the pain.

9. **While it currently isn't legal to use MAiD for mental illness, that expansion is anticipated to be put into effect March 17, 2027.**

   Unless there are major improvements in the healthcare system before then, it may feel like the logical option/solution when so much of living with a disability involves fighting for the necessary supports to keep living.

To be very clear, I respect each person's sovereignty over their bodies and do not wish to remove that. However, I recognize some people respond to overwhelm with suicidal ideations, and there are a variety of social pressures that leave people with disabilities (especially newly disabled individuals) in disordered mental states, considering options they normally wouldn't. I know multiple people who survived suicide attempts, and the ones I've discussed things with are grateful their attempt failed.

I feel allowing for assisted suicide is a bad idea due to the severity of societal ableism (which pushes disabled people towards poverty), ageism (which devalues the life of elderly people), and classism (which devalues the lives of poor people). If and when those issues are managed, I'm happy to discuss the right of an individual to choose to end their own life or have assistance to do so.

Until then, I think we need to focus on the reasons why people contemplate death and improve their quality of life so that poverty and ableism do not have the kind of power they currently do.

Abortion and Eugenics

Abortion is healthcare, and the decision to keep or terminate a pregnancy is one that should be made by the parent/s with advice from their doctor. In the disability community, we are often in the awkward position of being used as arguments both for and against abortion rights. I want to be very clear, I oppose making abortions illegal or difficult to obtain. I want all pregnant people able to have an abortion if they determine it's the necessary or appropriate course of action. I believe putting many limits on that right is immoral.

 **ICELAND**

Actions do have consequences though, and we need to be aware of the impact ableism can have on these decisions. For example, the country of Iceland has encouraged genetic testing and discouraged the birth of children with Down Syndrome to such a degree that there are almost no children in that country with the condition[45].

Down Syndrome impacts a child and the adult that they grow up to become, but it isn't a condition that in itself causes low quality of life. Decisions based on genetic imperfection is a deeply morally gray area and one that needs to be discussed and considered, but those details are beyond the scope of this volume.

I do feel it's important to be aware that abortion is a very complex topic within the disability community, and respect and nuance are vital in these conversations and considerations. Are there some conditions that should have an abortion rate approaching 100%? Possibly. However, not all disabilities are so terrible that the potential child should always be aborted if they have the potential to have a disability.

Eugenics and IVF

Historically, the fertility of disabled people has been controlled at times by abled people in positions of power. The practice of eugenics (improving the genetic quality of the human population by reducing or removing the fertility of "undesirable" or "inferior" portions of the population) has always had more severe disabilities in its crosshairs, and regularly used disability as their underlying argument of that inferiority (we discussed this in earlier chapters).

From concentration camps during World War II to forced sterilizations of mentally ill or "severely disabled" people (especially women), there is a long history of using disability as the stated reason for sterilizing or killing people to improve the "purity" of the human race.

---

45 Rugaard, Sophie. "Iceland appears to have virtually eliminated Down syndrome through abortion." CBS News. Published August 15, 2017. Accessed April 10, 2025. **https://www.cbsnews.com/news/down-syndrome-iceland/**.

With capitalism, most of our value to society is financial, and as we've discussed, people with disabilities are regularly pushed towards or into poverty, which, combined with ableism, both reduces our options in partners (high divorce rates, etc.) and reduces the number of children we can responsibly choose to have. It increases the risk of children we do have being traumatized, poorly educated, and less employable, all of which reduces their options for success.

This discussion isn't complete without mentioning IVF (In Vitro Fertilization), which can create emotionally problematic situations.

For example, there are many disabilities caused by genetic imperfections that IVF professionals screen for. This means that parents with disabilities who use IVF can be prevented from having children who share their disabilities (see resources). This can cause mixed feelings to say the least.

There are arguments in every direction related to this. Intentionally creating a generation of disabled individuals is absolutely a morally gray area, especially with the severity of ableism in the world.

Some people who identify as "pro-life" (though it's really "pro-birth", since many of these people are opposed to most social welfare programs) have issues with IVF since it necessarily includes fertilizing eggs with no intention of ever implanting them in a womb. In the meantime, IVF is an extremely expensive process, so is only available to people who can afford it.

As genetic information becomes more detailed, we run more of a risk of having an abled, "genetically superior" class of people, children of the wealthy people who could afford genetic screening and manipulation of their potential offspring.

Is this an immediate threat? Maybe not, but on the path society is heading down, it is a risk, and one we're seeing the potential of through things like Iceland's work to prevent the birth of people with Down Syndrome.

I am not morally opposed to IVF technology or some degree of genetic manipulation of potential humans. I simply think it's important to recognize the potential ramifications of this technology becoming widely used on the larger disability community.

Awareness of our right to exist

I wrote this chapter because I strongly feel we as disabled people need to understand our history better to help avoid repeating the mistakes of the past. Recognizing how deep ableism runs in society helps us put our struggles into perspective and helps us recognize historical threats when they take new, updated, more subtle forms.

We are fully human, and we deserve to exist and be treated with respect. Recognizing the ways, times, and places where that has not been true helps us push back against misinformation, educate ourselves and others, and take the necessary steps to protect ourselves in a society that is not designed for us and has not consistently recognized our humanity.

These are some of the costs our ancestors, relatives, and fellow disabled folks have paid, and continue to pay, so the least we can do is witness it and protect the next generation of disabled folks from the worst of these fates.

KEY POINTS

- People with disabilities are at higher risk of losing their **reproductive rights** or abilities (sterilization), or of being targeted for **abuse, neglect** or **death** by their government.

- Some countries have discussed **euthanasia** for severely disabled citizens, especially those whose diagnoses are terminal and likely to be extremely painful. Structural ableism makes this conversation much more fraught and increases the risk of death for people who could have high quality lives if their government provided appropriate support in a reasonable time frame.

- **Abortion** is **medical care**, but **ableism** can lead to disproportionate termination of pregnancies where the fetus is **diagnosed** with a condition that doesn't mean lower quality of life (e.g., Iceland's termination of most pregnancies that would lead to children with Down Syndrome).

- **IVF** practices include rules against implanting embryos with certain genetic imperfections, which means that disabled parents using these practices can be prevented from having children who share their diagnosis.

RESOURCES

"Medical assistance in dying." Health Canada. Last modified March 28, 2024. Accessed April 10, 2025. **https://www.canada.ca/en/health-canada/services/health-services-benefits/medical-assistance-dying.html**.

Flores, Marie E.S. 2024. "My Journey to Motherhood: A Parenting Odyssey." In **Disability Intimacy: Essays on Love, Care, and Desire**, edited by Alice Wong. New York: Vintage Books. Marie used IVF and had multiple eggs considered unusable because they shared her disability.

RESOURCES WEBPAGE » CHAPTER 11

CHAPTER 12

Citizenship, Immigration, and Disability
No country wants more disabled citizens

With the United States of America's 2024 election results and the responses to it top of mind, I want to recognize a simple fact: NO country wants disabled citizens.

Most countries have created barriers to entry for the average citizen of another country, and very often those barriers explicitly or implicitly prevent people with disabilities from becoming citizens or long-term residents of their country.

Every conversation I've had related to travel between countries, and every bit of research I have done has included that the country you wish to move to needs proof of sustainable income (or assets) above a certain level (basically enough to comfortably support yourself so your presence is a net gain for their economy) and/or having a skill or skillset that's in high demand (often both). Exceptions are made if you marry a citizen or are sponsored by a citizen, but there still is often an expectation of being or becoming a wage-earning member of society whose income keeps you above needing their social safety net.

People who are on most disability support programs cannot do these things. Our conditions prevent us from earning our country's definition of substantial income, and our social welfare programs (if we are eligible for them) generally provide support on the very low end of our country's acceptable pay spectrum.

As all social welfare systems of today are set up, a citizen with any type of disability can only succeed if they are above-average in multiple other respects, able to overcome the biases of the medical system, education system (which we'll discuss in Chapter 13), and employment system, and be able to do so despite the structural barriers that are in play to prevent their participation in society. That is a lot to overcome. Some people absolutely do manage to do so, but it isn't easy.

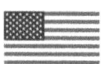 **UNITED STATES OF AMERICA**

Another thing to be aware of is that the US is especially ableist when it comes to immigration.

I had a conversation about this with an American who is married to an Austrian. When she moved to Austria with him, no medical exams were required, but when he moved to the US with her, he had to undergo a medical examination as part of his screening process. This implies if he'd been "too disabled", he could have been denied entry to the US or denied a path to citizenship.

 **AUSTRIA**

Austria, at least, did not require medical information to decide on a citizen's spouse's citizenship.

It isn't just the United States who uses health and healthcare as part of their decision-making process.

 NEW ZEALAND

New Zealand had a long-running controversy over a family who immigrated from South Africa. The wife was overweight and that was used to deny her family citizenship[46].

While she eventually was allowed to become a citizen (and her family did stay in New Zealand despite the challenges and publicity), her primary point throughout much of the fight was that in her case she was healthy, and so not particularly likely to become a drain on the system, rather than the route of pointing out the ableism inherent in the government refusing to grant citizenship based on her weight in the first place.

All systems have cracks you can slip through

If you are reading this series hoping for ideas on countries that might be better to live in as a person with disabilities (and I'm sure many of us have fantasized about moving somewhere better), I want you to be sure to do your homework, and realize that even if citizens are treated better in this other country that does NOT guarantee that you, as a non-citizen, will be.

I discussed laws in other countries with several Americans who had moved into European systems, and one of them shared the health insurance issues she and her spouse had experienced while living in a country with socialized medicine.

The systems aren't necessarily what Americans may assume and as a non-citizen, you are especially likely to miss an essential step, to be held responsible for failure to meet a certain burden of proof, or simply to not be eligible for any specific service because your situation is relatively unique. There is always the potential for bad actors in terms of employment (or simply misunderstandings of the law in regard to employment) so if you are working (or if you stop working), you may not qualify for the protections presumed to be in place.

---

46   Gill, Sinead "Too Fat for NZ: Mum Can't Lose Weight Fast Enough for Immigration Officials." Stuff. **https://www.stuff.co.nz/national/health/300341891/too-fat-for-nz-mum-cant-lose-weight-fast-enough-for-immigration-officials**.

For example, all European nations have single-payer healthcare in some form or another. However, that does not mean everyone is covered by exactly the same insurance. Many countries may have different government agencies responsible for coverage depending on your age or employment status.

 **AUSTRIA**

Austria, for example, has one coverage for people who have an employer, a different coverage for unemployed people, and yet another coverage for people who choose to be self-employed. Each has a payment program that is related to taxes, but the sources, people covered, and detailed rules of the coverage are different.

This means it's possible to be dropped from coverage by one, but that doesn't guarantee another program immediately picks up your coverage. For example, a person whose employment hours drop may get shuttled between barely qualifying for the employment-based coverage (due to number of hours worked) or being financially on the high end of the unemployment eligibility (due to not working enough hours to qualify for employment-based coverage).

Make sure you do your research!

As a community, disabled people often find ourselves on the margins of society's definitions, and generally in need of more support from our governments than the average (abled) person. This makes it essential, if we're considering any major life change, to look through the lens of our disability needs.

If you are seriously considering immigrating to any other country, look into their legal protections for people with disabilities. Check their healthcare laws and understand if and how you could become eligible for their benefit programs, healthcare coverage, and legal protections.

Talk to people who live in that country about how your symptoms, treatment options, and accessibility needs are (or aren't) met, and take the time to really understand if or how your protections in your home country might or might not help you. I want to be very clear, I am not discouraging you from looking into your options, I simply want to make sure you don't make assumptions about coverage that turn out to be untrue.

This is also true if you take medications and plan on traveling over a longer period of time than you would easily bring medicine for. Wherever you decide to travel, understand what the rules are in terms of you being able to fill your prescriptions, and what (if any) insurance will cover it.

I have heard stories from friends in other countries about folks who didn't plan and were hit with some very expensive lessons. Use common sense and make sure that you know what it would take to replace anything you lose or need to replace while traveling, including refilling any medications you take, or maintenance work for any accessibility tools you might have or need. Especially given how often wheelchairs are damaged by airlines[47,] you want to have a plan in place in case your mobility aid or other accessibility tool is damaged or lost in transit.

I want to direct your attention to a couple of disabled bloggers I know as they both have useful experiences and information resources for disabled folks who are considering travel or experiencing other parts of the world. My friend Carrie Kellenberger is Canadian and lives in Taiwan with her American husband. Her blog, **My Several Worlds**, contains a lot of valuable information about her experiences, including how she has navigated the Taiwanese medical system as a Canadian expat.

I also want to mention Sheryl Chan, who has been very active within the disability blogging community. She lives in Singapore and is native to that country but has made a point of collecting stories from other disabled folks, including encouraging people to share information on just how accessible (or inaccessible) their home city and country are based on their experiences. Her blog helps reinforce the similarities of our experiences as people with disabilities, and her section specifically focused on accessibility could be an amazing guide to help you understand the challenges you are likely to meet wherever you consider moving to (or for you to share tips on your city or country to help other disabled people considering moving or visiting there).

---

47   Morris, John. "Checking in on Wheelchair Damage: How Airlines Are Doing." *Wheelchair Travel*, October 25, 2023. **https://wheelchairtravel.org/airline-wheelchair-damage-statistics-update-october-2023/**

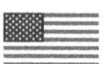 **UNITED STATES OF AMERICA**

You can travel while collecting SSDI, traveling on SSI is harder.

If the idea of being a digital nomad appeals to you, technically that is something you could do while collecting SSDI benefits. If you maintain a home address in the US and choose to travel, even for months at a time, your benefits will continue.

You may face challenges getting access to healthcare or managing your medication, but those are things you may be able to plan around or create solutions for. Of course, your options while traveling may be limited due to your disability itself, or your finances, but you could, in theory, meander your way around the world, taking time to manage your health while doing so.

Trying to do something similar while managing SSI benefits would be much more challenging though, as that program's rules state that your coverage is suspended if you are out of the country for more than 30 days.

When it comes to insurance, more challenges become obvious, but again carefully timed trips back to the US may help you manage at least some of those challenges.

SSDI and Medicare coverage protect you consistently no matter where in the US you are, so traveling within the US is (in theory) a viable option. People supported by SSI, on the other hand, would have a harder time traveling outside of their local area for more than a few days or weeks as their health insurance (Medicaid) is unlikely to be honored outside their home state.

KEY POINTS

- **No country wants more disabled citizens**. If you are thinking about moving to another country, or traveling long-term, make sure you understand the laws and attitudes in that country related to your disability, medical needs, and medications, and what services you may or may not be eligible for wherever you travel.

- People on SSDI can (in theory) travel to other countries for at least months at a time, but if you are on SSI, leaving the country for more than a month will result in your benefits being suspended.

RESOURCES

Kellenberger, Carrie. "My Several Worlds - Chronic Illness and Disability in Asia." My Several Worlds, April 3, 2025. **https://www.myseveralworlds.com/**

Chan, Sheryl. "Invisible Cities Linkup: Pros & Cons Of Living With Chronic Illness In Your City." A Chronic Voice, September 14, 2018. **https://www.achronicvoice.com/2018/09/14/invisible-cities-linkup/**

Hayes, Alison. "Can You Travel While On Disability?" Thriving While Disabled, August 10, 2018. **https://thrivingwhiledisabled.com/can-you-travel-while-on-disability/**

RESOURCES WEBPAGE » CHAPTER 12

CHAPTER 13

Education and Disability

In our increasingly complex society, education is becoming more and more vital for our ability to participate in everything our world has to offer. As people with disabilities, many of us have or will find ourselves struggling to get the education we deserve.

Whether our disabilities are apparent or non-apparent, many of us can struggle with the social environments of our schools, as well as the rigid structures often involved in attending.

Like most minority identities, our stories generally are not told in school, and like others who are different, we may well experience various forms of "othering" including bullying, bias, and intolerance.

Our differences often require schools themselves to make changes or adjustments to accommodate us, and structural ableism is again apparent in the design of the school and curriculum.

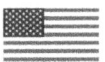 **UNITED STATES OF AMERICA**

In the US, disabled students are now protected, but that has been the case for less than 50 years. The right to be educated is supposed to be legally protected as part of our civil rights internationally, but every country, including the US, is variable in just how strongly they enforce that expectation and what protections they have in place.

NEW ZEALAND

For example, New Zealand schools in 2020 still illegally prevented almost one third of disabled students from participating in school.[48] This was an improvement from prior studies, where closer to forty percent of students were prevented. Disabled students who attended often were educated by professionals who felt underprepared for working with students with their needs.

 GLOBAL

Normalizing disability is a vital part of combating ableism, and we tend to be more mentally flexible as children. This makes it all the more important for children with disabilities to actively participate in classes and get the same educational opportunities as abled children.

The more exposure children have to the diversity of our societies, the more adaptable they will be to future changes. Disability representation matters, and an essential part of that, one of the keys to breaking down ableism, is to have children with disabilities fully participate in education and the school community.

Take a few minutes and think about your experiences in school. Were you a disabled student? Did you have a classmate with a disability? Was disability discussed?

I know we had a class or two discussing Helen Keller, but they were primarily focused on her disabled identity (a deaf-blind woman who learned to communicate), rather than on her activism or politics.

As a community, we need to be educated and have our participation normalized. That means schools should be fully accessible, barrier-free, and follow universal design principles (we discuss those further in Chapter 19). They should have educational supports for children with disabilities built into their curriculum and educational plans.

---

48 New Zealand Herald. 2024. "Appalling: Almost One in Three Children with Disabilities Unlawfully Denied School Enrolment." NZ Herald. **https://www.nzherald.co.nz/nz/appalling-almost-one-in-threechildren-with-disabilities-unlawfully-denied-school-enrolment/ KPRYXQZ5V2WYFTSWZICHHWNLWU/**

Your disabled child's right to an education

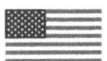 **UNITED STATES OF AMERICA**

US CHILDREN'S EDUCATIONAL RIGHTS AT-A-GLANCE

Eligibility:
- All children in the US are guaranteed free, appropriate education in the least restrictive environment possible.
- Annual Individual Education Plans (IEPs) should be created every year for each disabled student to ensure they have and are meeting appropriate educational milestones.
- Section 504 (of the Architectural Barriers Act - Accessibility) rights focus on their ability to participate in school and community activities.

Checking your eligibility:
- Your disabled child is eligible for support through the Department of Education from birth (or start of disabling symptoms).

What information they need:
- Proof of residency (so they know what municipality, county, and state needs to provide resources).
- Proof (or indicators) of your child's disability.
- You do not need a diagnosis, but you need enough information to indicate what type/s of testing, evaluation, or support your child might need.
- Accommodations your child needs (often this is initially determined through an evaluation).

Where do you apply?
- Individual supports will vary, but **https://www.ed.gov/laws-and-policy/individuals-disabilities/idea** is a good place to start. Specialty programs may need to be applied for individually based upon your child's needs and what is available in your area.

When do you apply?

- As soon as you are aware your child has a disability. If they show signs of developmental delays or are dealing with physical differences, contact your local school district (if your child is 5 or over) or social services (if your child is younger).

How long does it take?

- Depends on needs and on your local support network. Some support provided may overlap with options provided by health insurance (so you have options for testing, evaluation, or treatment), other support may overlap with social welfare supports, and still other services may be unique.

How long does it last?

- Children are eligible for support through the Department of Education until they age out at 21 years of age.
- Individualized Education Plans (IEP)s should be discussed at least annually with teachers K-12.
- Accommodations (if needed) should be discussed at least annually.

Who do I talk to if things go wrong?

- Your school district is your initial and primary point of contact. Most will have a social worker, counselor, or other designated special education department representative. Generally, you should be given that information early in the process of getting your child's needs met. The contact person may change annually or whenever your child changes schools.
- If you feel your child's rights are being violated, you may be able to make others in the school system or social welfare system aware. If that effort is unsuccessful, reach out to your county or state government for further support (the process is discussed in Volume II). You may reach out to the federal Department of Education for enforcement.

How many students are disabled?

In the US, about 15% of students (7.5 million 2022–2023 school year) are recognized as disabled, and 32% of them have learning disabilities[49]. Despite about 2.4 million students in the US school system having documented learning disabilities, universal design in learning is not yet widely embraced.

All children who need Special Education Support in public school have the legal right to an IEP (Individualized Education Plan), which describes what adjustments will be made to work with their disabilities and what their educational goals are for the year. There generally is pressure to keep children with others the same age, and so some children (especially those with disabilities) are at risk of continuing to go up to the next grade level even if they haven't mastered (or in some cases, understood) age-appropriate subjects. By going over your child's IEP, you are doing your best to hold the school responsible for educating your child, rather than simply providing childcare.

All children with a disability that impacts one or more life activities legally have the right for a 504 (Accessibility) Plan, which allows them to participate in class alongside their peers. Look at the 504 Plan as the way your child is able to interact with peers and teachers, participate in school events and opportunities, and be part of the school community.

The quality of support services, testing, 504 Plans, and IEPs (and how well progress is measured) can and will vary dramatically among school districts. Generally speaking, schools in more affluent areas will have better support for students with disabilities. They often have fewer students with disabilities, as many disabilities are associated with poverty (as we've discussed in Chapter 4).

---

[49] National Center for Education Statistics. *The Condition of Education, 2024*.
https://nces.ed.gov/programs/coe/pdf/2024/CGG_508c.pdf

GLOBAL

Disabled children's education rights in your country

One of the many ways ableism impacts the world is through educational opportunities and their lack. In the global north, children are expected to participate in their country's education system until they are legally considered adults, or until completing the publicly mandated curriculum. While disabled children are technically expected to do these things, many countries either fail to enforce these rules with certain children with disabilities, or they actively deny entry to school for children with certain disabilities. Students with learning disabilities need their school to provide educational material in a different way than abled students, which again occurs to varying degrees.

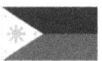 **PHILIPPINES**

In the global south, things can be even worse. I had an amazing conversation with a woman in the Philippines who was prevented from attending school by the school administration because, as a blind student, they feared that her classmates would be more focused on her than on their lessons. The teachers freely admitted that they had no idea how to teach a blind student. No attempts were made to accommodate her or normalize her disability, and her parents accepted this out of their own fears for her safety. From our conversation, I gleaned she was relatively fortunate as other children with disabilities were effectively abandoned by their families due to fear, superstition, or lack of resources.

She shared that it was easier for people to not think about their children with disabilities and ignore their needs than to fight for their rights, accommodations, and care. Her sense of things, which I wholeheartedly agree with, is the issue at its most basic is one of education. There are ways to teach students with disabilities, and there are ways to manage most disabling conditions. But people need to have their basic needs met and allocate resources towards understanding how disabilities work, and how to create more accessible spaces so disabled children can fully participate in society too.

If the area you live in is struggling to get students to school or to provide textbooks or teachers, then your disabled child is likely to be forgotten, ignored, or pushed out. If your country, county, or community is generally wealthier, and your area is generally more accessible, there's a greater chance of a disabled child getting a quality education. But I would anticipate, no matter where you live, you're going to have to struggle more and fight harder for your child to have a good education than your peers with abled children.

As in other areas of life, society has a bias towards supporting children who fit the normative model for education and against making adjustments to that model, even when (or if) the adjustment is proven to be more effective.

It's useful to know there has been a good amount of research into educational models to help students with and without disabilities learn better and more effectively. This is called the **universal design for learning**, and while it has not been fully embraced anywhere, it could be an incredible tool for you to advocate for your school to adopt or at least use with your child (or children). The better you understand your child's needs and diagnosis, the better you can argue for the appropriate supports for them in school.

National laws saying children need to be educated are often in conflict with local realities, so you want to understand your child's rights and your local school system's limitations before they are of age to attend school if at all possible.

When it comes to the transition from childhood to adulthood and protections in regard to a college education, I can only share what I've learned and experienced within the US.

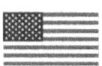 UNITED STATES OF AMERICA

Be aware the current political conversations about defunding the Department of Education would have a profoundly negative impact on disabled children, as much of the funding for and enforcement of their full participation in their school district comes directly from the Federal Department of Education. Local school districts, especially poorer ones, would not be able to make up for the financial shortfalls. Without the federal DOE to enforce regulations, the likelihood of local school districts failing to enforce student disability protections skyrockets.

Brief history of disabled children's education rights in the US

Children with disabilities were not guaranteed the right to attend public school until 1975. Attending public school was considered compulsory (required) in 34 states in 1900, and compulsory in all states for abled children up to the age of 14 in 1930. During this time, most children with intellectual or severe physical or psychiatric disabilities were institutionalized.

Into and through the 1940s, polio was one of the larger mass disabling events, with swaths of children contracting the disease and the survivors becoming physically disabled. Many of the children who survived would get to know one another through regular or long-term hospitalizations and social networks of adults who had become disabled as children grew, often pushing for increased rights and access for disabled people. In the meantime, other networks of parents of disabled children (especially those with intellectual and developmental disabilities) started gathering.

1954's end to school segregation by race was part of a new era of social change. Groups of parents of disabled children started pushing local and eventually federal governments to allow their children to attend school and get the education that was required for abled children.

By 1955, Jonas Salk had created a vaccine for polio that Americans were eager to share, greatly reducing the rate of disability and death due to polio. Other vaccines were created during this time, increasing survival rates of additional diseases. Slowly, more and more local governments made the adjustments required to allow children with physical or intellectual disabilities to attend school, and slowly the federal government passed individual laws that protected some of those children's rights.

By 1970, 1 in 5 children with disabilities were educated in US public schools, while many states still had laws actively excluding deaf, blind, emotionally disturbed, or intellectually disabled children.

The Individuals with Disabilities Education Act (originally Education for all Handicapped Children Act) was passed by President Gerald Ford in 1975. It guarantees free, appropriate, public education in the least restrictive environment possible to all children with disabilities.

While the original laws covered children aged from kindergarten to 12th grade, the modern IDEA (the name was changed in 1990 when the ADA was passed) provides protection and transition support for disabled individuals birth-21, with a greater focus on holding educators responsible for meeting general education requirements. As of the 2022-2023 school year, IDEA is supporting over 8 million children (birth-21) with disabilities.

The goal for students with disabilities is for all to receive free appropriate public education, including continuing their education opportunities through the age of 21 when appropriate.

My experiences as a Special Education student

My early experiences predate the ADA.

I was fortunate enough to be evaluated for developmental delays through a program created by a local university (so their students could experience giving the appropriate testing), where they found I had gross motor (limb and body control) limitations. My mom and I were given exercises to do to help improve control of my body, and by the time I started kindergarten I primarily only had issues with fine motor control (primarily hands). The school I attended had a "resource room" (which fellow students described with a much less pleasant "r" word) where I was sent one class period a day for support. I had accommodations, which in my case included typing notes in class (very unusual in the 80s), and extra time on tests.

My father taught me to type when I was about 6 specifically so I'd be able to use a keyboard, and my parents provided me with a predecessor of a laptop, which was a very small 4-line screen above a full-sized keyboard (I do not know whether they or the school purchased it or if there was some kind of cost split). I was very fortunate, both that my parents were able to advocate for me and make those accommodations happen, and that we lived in a well-funded school district willing to provide quality services.

I was in the more advanced reading and math classes, scored in the 99th percentile in most standardized testing, but wasn't invited to participate in my school's gifted and talented program because the school wasn't prepared for a student with both deficits and strengths, only the more typical "straight A" type student.

> I think I had IEPs every year, which is what allowed the accommodations to continue. I was around 12 years old when the ADA was passed, and I was aware I was getting learning accommodations. I was occasionally bullied for the various ways I was different (less socially aware than classmates, attending the resource room, in the advanced classes, things like that), but I didn't identify as disabled. The word just didn't click as describing me, even though I knew I had a learning disability and was struggling off and on with depression.
>
> When I attended high school, I was in and out of the top-tier classes, taking the occasional Honors/AP class, and some classes simply labeled as "college prep". Overall, I was a good, but not great, student, generally understanding the concepts quickly, but regularly making what my teachers referred to as "careless errors".

Recognizing the power and limitations of Disability protections for students

The key term throughout this entire section is "public". These are the laws, rules, and expectations for public schools. Private schools do not receive government funding and so aren't held to many of these laws or standards. While it's possible that some private schools may try to follow some of these as recommendations, there are no legal protections, and they can't be held legally liable for not providing these supports.

This is one of the many reasons why the discussions in the US about school vouchers is a disability issue. A national voucher program would take money earmarked for a public school, which is legally required to be accessible, and give it to a private school, which isn't.

When parents are paying for their child to attend a private school, their tax dollars are still being paid towards the public school in their community. The census calculations are unchanged, so the Department of Education is providing the same amount of funding to the schools. The public school is still getting all the funding it is legally entitled to in order to keep supporting all students. One less student in the classrooms doesn't change much for the school system, but the dollars attached to that student might, especially when multiplied over the 12-plus years they're anticipated to attend school.

If we passed the voucher system nationally (some states have passed vouchers in some form), every child that attended private school could (depending on how the law was written) remove money earmarked for the public school, leaving the school with less funding than it otherwise would have received. Because our school systems are already struggling financially, the schools would need to cut their budgets even further, likely increasing class size and reducing the money available for "extras".

As we've discussed previously, accessibility and other disability needs already are usually considered "extra" in the grand scheme of things, so the most likely cuts would be to either the maintenance of equipment (including those necessary for accessibility), delays in repairs to equipment (including those needed for accessibility), or reduction in staffing or staff education (which often includes support staff or bias education). The other likely cuts could involve testing for learning disabilities, support for students with learning disabilities, or other things that decrease how easy or accessible it is to have children tested for or proved in need of supports from the school system. If there's no documented need, then support isn't legally required.

We have a great disparity in education in the US due to the racist, classist, and ableist practice of funding public education through property taxes. Public schools are already struggling financially, and the programs designed to help combat that (additional funding by the federal government for low-income school districts) has not done enough to correct these issues.

All students deserve a quality education, and unfortunately disabled students are one of many populations still not consistently receiving one.

Parents: Helping your disabled child transition to adulthood

If you have a disabled child who is approaching adulthood, or you are a young disabled adult, you'll have noticed many programs specifically differentiate between childhood and adulthood, with different rules for each. The age of adulthood varies, but 18 and 21 are the two most commonly referenced ages in the US. So, what exactly is the transition point and what happens during it?

Depending on state and federal law, a person is legally considered an adult at the age of 18 (for example, voting) or 21 (for example, alcohol consumption). A disabled child is eligible for SSI coverage as a child as long as they are under 18. From that point, they are considered under the adult guidelines, which are different.

When a person has a disability, most activities follow those of their abled peers, but there are a few special cases.

When it comes to education, for example, most people are expected to graduate from high school around the age of 18, which is the end of the legal expectation that they attend school. Students with disabilities, however, may attend schooling and be supported by IDEA until the age of 21, so their families have some time to help them transition from the standard education system to their next step in life.

This may include some form of vocational training, continuing their high school education, support services towards independent employment, moving into some form of supportive housing, or other possibilities.

This gives the parent/s (who in the case of certain developmental or intellectual disabilities may be the primary decision maker/s for the rest of their lives) some time to figure out next steps or apply for appropriate support programs before funding support ends. Some parents consider this age range to be a time of approaching a cliff, since their child will no longer be eligible for many of the supports the parents are familiar with, and there is no longer much focus by support programs on their child's growth and development.

Since adulthood is commonly viewed by society as the time when a person shifts from being an expense, someone to educate and mold, to a producer, somebody who works and earns money, ableism and classism tend to make everything about the transition to adulthood for people who have never worked and cannot be expected to work especially dark and daunting.

If you are living with your child, and plan to have them continue to live with you, they still can receive SSI benefits (as long as they fit adult eligibility rules), though you may wish to investigate if it makes sense to help them be legally considered a separate household. While that doesn't have to happen immediately, it may be a way to help them have a better sense of independence, something that can be especially challenging when living with a disability.

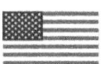 **UNITED STATES OF AMERICA**

Disabled Adult Child Benefits

The period between 18 and 21 allows disabled individuals to apply for SSI benefits if their parents' income was too high for eligibility previously and marks the earliest point of eligibility for DAC (Disabled Adult Child) benefits.

Disabled Adult Child benefits are specifically for people who became too disabled to work before the age of 22. The other prerequisite is that at least one of that person's parents must be (or have been) eligible for Social Security benefits. I recently worked with a client whose SSI benefits started when they were 23, though they had never actively worked full time. Unfortunately, they were unable to get DAC coverage because while they were too disabled to work at 22, Social Security does not have that on record and will not backdate their onset of disability date. I'm sharing this here in hopes of protecting you from experiencing the same problem.

What are DAC benefits? They allow the adult child of a person eligible for SSDI to also collect SSDI benefits (including Medicare), when their parent retires or passes away, for the rest of that adult child's life. This is basically one of the very few ways to "double-dip" into Social Security funds. While the child does not get the full amount, they do receive 50-75% of what their highest-earning parent receives (or received).

I'll give you a real-life example.

I have a family member who is a DAC recipient. He became disabled at the age of 20 and eventually received SSI coverage (and therefore Medicaid coverage, etc.). When his father retired, both of them became Medicare eligible and both of them started receiving a monthly check from Social Security. His father receives the full amount (his retirement benefits), and the adult child receives his percentage (through DAC). My relative will receive that check and keep the eligibility for the rest of his life. He will remain eligible for both Medicare and Medicaid for that same period.

The logic of it is that the parent has been caring for their adult disabled child for that child's entire life. Now the parent can no longer work, they are no longer held financially responsible for their child's support and can have the peace of mind of knowing that their child will be cared for for the rest of their life.

My relative's father has created a Special Needs trust for him, which will hold his inheritance. By creating the Special Needs Trust, the father has protected his child from potentially losing Medicaid/SSI eligibility when he passes away.

If you or your child has the potential to be eligible for DAC coverage, make sure their documented onset of disability date (discussed in Volume II) is before their 22nd birthday!

Planning for college with a Disability

At this age, your child (or you, if you are the child in question) may be looking to attend college. If so, you probably want to focus with them on finding an accessible college (one that has a good reputation for accessibility standards), and if appropriate, helping them do so in a state with a good Home and Community-Based Care program (Medicaid) that meets their needs.

If they need a personal care assistant (for example), living in a state that allows them to hire one of their own may both give them more independence and allow them to feel more empowered.

When I went to college, my accessibility needs were relatively simple, but I remember even then there were guidebooks that discussed colleges that were more (or less) friendly to accessibility requests and differences in learning styles. When you (or you and your child) look into colleges, you will want to investigate the appropriate details for their/your disability.

> **A family member who experienced a brain injury in high school, ended up attending multiple colleges due in part to structural ableism.**
>
> Initially, she attended our local community college to give herself more recovery time. This went relatively well.
>
> The first four-year institution she then went to was very inflexible, which led to her changing schools again.
>
> Red flag #1 was they assumed that everyone would graduate in four years and placed a huge emphasis on doing things by your anticipated graduating class.
>
> They weren't thrilled with her having attended community college first, and were even more negative about the idea she would need to take a half-time course load per semester due to her disability. Their disability services department left a lot to be desired.
>
> When she did transfer out, her new college had an excellent disability services department, which cheerfully met her needs and exceeded her expectations. For example, she needed her textbooks for classes to be in large print.
>
> The first school gave her access to a photocopier that would enlarge the text (expecting her to do the rest). The second school took her books before the school term began, made the large print copies, and spiral-bound the material together so she'd have an actual textbook she could read and use. If I remember correctly, I believe they divided some of the books into multiple bound sections, so they'd be easier to carry with her and gave her a standard-sized copy of some of the books as well in case she needed them.

If you live in a state with a Home and Community-Based Care program (discussed in Volume II) that allows the disabled individual to hire their own PCA, and your child plans on continuing to live with you (or you as the disabled individual plans to continue to live with your parents), you may want to apply for the PCA program as well, since it would allow the disabled individual to pay for in-home services and keep more money in the home (or allow the disabled individual to hire a friend and relieve their parents of some of those duties).

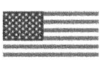 **UNITED STATES OF AMERICA**

Legal protections in college

Generally, college students are legally adults and are no longer primarily provided legal protections by the Department of Education. This means that IDEA protections no longer apply, but the Section 504 laws still do.

For higher education, buildings are legally expected to be physically accessible, but because so little attention is paid to compliance, it's quite possible many facilities aren't, or the administration describes them as accessible, but they aren't as accessible as implied.

Colleges and Universities are legally expected to be physically accessible, according to laws by both the Department of Education and the Architectural Barriers Act, but sometimes the only way to ensure that they are accessible is through lawsuit.

If you don't want to be a trailblazer, visit the campus in advance to see if it meets your accessibility needs. Both laws are more focused on enforcement at public universities, so those are more likely to be more accessible, but many private colleges and universities have received some form of government funding at some point and are likely to be at least somewhat accessible.

When it comes to learning disabilities or other non-apparent conditions, it's a bit trickier to evaluate in advance. Most, if not all, colleges have some form of Disability Services department and you will want to talk to them in advance, both so they can help you plan a visit, and possibly to help you weed out poor options.

While some Disability Services departments are great, others leave a lot to be desired, and it's quite possible these departments will be more skilled with some types of disabilities than others. You want to feel confident that the Disability Services department is ready, willing, and able to go to bat for you and understands your needs well.

My Disability Service experiences

I had experience personally with two different Disability Services departments when I went to school, one for college and the other for graduate school.

In college, I needed accommodations for my learning disabilities, in the form of untimed exams, taking my exams outside the classroom (usually in an empty room nearby) and use of my computer for note and test-taking (I can type much more quickly, neatly, and effectively than hand write things).

I needed to provide an evaluation by an appropriate education professional showing my need for these supports (the first time that had been requested in my case), but that was about it. Each term, they would send notifications of this need to all my professors, and my request was honored.

I only had one professor who ever questioned it, and he and I had a conversation about how we could best meet my needs. It turned out he was only concerned about two aspects of fairness: he was a philosophy professor, and his essay exams were intended to be graded without him knowing which student turned them in. He was concerned about my turning in printed out documents interfering with that anonymity and that giving extra time would prevent part of his goal of having us work within time constraints.

We ended up agreeing I would hold to the time limit, and he would do his best not to be unduly influenced by knowing who I was due to being the only student to hand in a typed paper.

I know I was extremely fortunate in this, as I've heard nightmare stories from many other disabled students. I suspect another component to this was I had chosen a small liberal arts college known for small class sizes and supportive professors. I absolutely acknowledge the privileges I had in education and family finances that allowed me to do this.

In graduate school, I was very fortunate. By then, I was living with my FND diagnosis, and so while my requests were similar, the logic was slightly different. Because my FND is stress-responsive, being in the classroom and feeling the pressure of the test being timed was likely to trigger my symptoms, and I wanted privacy in case I was symptomatic (both out of politeness of not wanting to distract my classmates and because the extra attention could worsen my symptoms and make recovery harder).

I requested flexibility on turning in assignments if my symptoms flared. Typing is still my easiest way to record my thoughts, and my handwriting becomes less legible the more quickly I write. Typing notes in class in the 2010s was, of course, much more common than it was in the late 1990s and early 2000s when I was in college, so that no longer required special permission, but it was still less common for exams (though most of my grad school classes had final papers rather than exams anyway). The major difference was instead of notifying my professors, they simply created a letter, which was updated each semester, that I was responsible for giving to my professors.

I again had few problems, but I made a point both in college and graduate school to approach my professors immediately following my first class with them, introducing myself and discussing my requests.

In college, this was to make sure they had been notified, and in graduate school, I was both confirming they'd received my email and preparing to discuss my FND symptoms with them. I always mentioned I had a movement disorder in my emails, but my symptoms can be a bit distracting, so I did my best to face it head on and explain that I couldn't prevent the movements, explain how broad my definition of "stress" was, and reassure them my symptoms weren't dangerous to me or others. I usually got positive responses. I made a point of explaining the request for extensions was due to symptoms and symptom flares, and I would do my best to notify them as far in advance as possible if I expected things to be delayed.

During graduate school I ended up experiencing multiple symptom flares, ended up needing to take multiple incompletes, and take a year off. I attended classes remotely multiple times, including for most of my final semester. My school worked with me, but I had again made a point of attending a graduate school with a relatively small program, and one with a focus on social justice.

Planning ahead can work wonders!

When preparing for college or graduate school, make sure you are aware of your needs and limitations, so you can clearly communicate them to the Disability Services program. When selecting a school, make sure they have a good Disability Services program that seems likely to work well with your specific needs.

It's much better to be disappointed on or when planning a college visit or deciding where to go, than it is to be disappointed when trying to start your first semester.

Ideally, you want to predominantly be worried about the same stuff as your classmates, not the extra stresses that come with being disabled—so the more you prepare in advance and the better research you do when planning where to go, the easier things will be when you start (and trust me, that's tough enough already!).

Check out the resources section for a link to guidance on college protections.

KEY POINTS

- In theory, **education** is mandatory for all children living in all countries, at least in the global north. In practice, children with disabilities are frequently "forgotten" by their local government.
- In the US, all children have the right to free, appropriate education in the least restrictive environment possible, as directed by IDEA (Individuals with Disabilities Education Act). The act covers children birth to 21 years of age.
- **Section 504** laws protect your child's right to physically access and participate in classroom, school, and community activities to the greatest extent possible.
- Your child should have an **Individualized Education Plan (IEP)** for K-12 education, which shows what they are expected to learn, and how the school will support their learning process.
- If your income is limited and/or your child's condition is severe, they may be eligible for **SSI** coverage starting after birth. If your household income or assets are too high, your child may be eligible for SSI coverage after they turn **18**. If their SSI coverage begins before the age of 22, they may be eligible for **Disabled Adult Child (DAC)** benefits.
- If your child is going to college (or you are preparing to attend college) make sure that the campus is accessible for them (you) and the school's disability services department can work well with their (your) needs.
- In college, students are protected by the Americans with Disability Act, and schools that receive funding from the Department of Education are expected to make their campuses accessible. Public schools are more likely to follow these laws than private ones, but as always, the degree of compliance can vary radically.

RESOURCES

Your child's right to an education

New Zealand Herald. 2024. "Appalling: Almost One in Three Children with Disabilities Unlawfully Denied School Enrolment." NZ Herald. **https://www.nzherald.co.nz/nz/appalling-almost-one-in-three-children-with-disabilities-unlawfully-denied-school-enrolment/KPRYXQZ5V2WYFTSWZICHHWNLWU/**.

Morin, Amanda. 2023. "Universal Design for Learning (UDL): What It Is and How It Works." Understood. **https://www.understood.org/en/articles/universal-design-for-learning-what-it-is-and-how-it-works**.

U.S. Department of Education. n.d. "Disability Discrimination: Providing a Free Appropriate Public Education (FAPE)." **https://www.ed.gov/laws-and-policy/civil-rights-laws/protecting-students/free-appropriate-public-education-fape**.

U.S. Department of Education. n.d. "Office of Special Education Programs (OSEP)." **https://www.ed.gov/about/ed-offices/osers/osep#OSEP-Programs-and-Projects.**

Programs directly provided by governmental bodies related to families with children with disabilities.

U.S. Department of Education. n.d. Individuals with Disabilities Education Act (IDEA) Topic Areas. Office of Special Education Programs. **https://sites.ed.gov/idea/topic-areas/**.

Example of College resource

BestColleges. n.d. "College Guide for Students with Disabilities." BestColleges. **https://www.bestcolleges.com/resources/students-with-disabilities/**.

13 » Education and Disability » **189**

RESOURCES WEBPAGE » CHAPTER 13

CHAPTER 14

Marriage
The financial and social realities

Many people assume that they are going to get married at some point. Marriage is an expected step in a person's life. It is painted as a net positive experience, with a focus on the advantages marriage brings. The possible disadvantages are rarely considered, and even more rarely mentioned.

In terms of employment, men are the ones who primarily benefit from being married, as employers view this as a valuable life step and proof of the man's reliability. Women do not get the same benefit, however, as employers assume marriage means children are on the horizon, which means maternity leave, extra days off work due to sick children, and other potential distractions from work life (yep, another example of sexism). Since women are often expected by society to change their last name, there are additional potential challenges to their professional lives with fewer benefits.

Having a disability may complicate the decision to get or not get married. Many support programs designed to help people with disabilities presume the disabled person they are helping is relatively poor. In many cases, if your household income is over a certain amount, you may not be eligible for certain types of assistance or you are eligible for less support than you otherwise would be. An unmarried person can argue they are a household of 1, even if they share certain expenses with others. A married person who shares living space with their spouse cannot.

GLOBAL

As I discuss the impact in the US, consider what might happen with your country's laws.

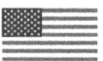 **UNITED STATES OF AMERICA**

Supplemental Security Income (SSI) has been called out by disability rights advocates, repeatedly and correctly, for what is referred to as their "marriage penalty" which is the most obvious way in which structural ableism influences marriage.

The financial cost of marriage on SSI

Most social welfare programs, including Supplemental Security Income (SSI), are based on financial need. As a single person, only your income and assets are considered in your application for these programs.

While SSI does provide some income to survive on, and SNAP benefits to help purchase food, the most important service SSI offers is Medicaid, which covers much, and sometimes all, of the medical needs of a person with a disability.

Those costs are the primary concern for a person with a disability, and if they are married, their spouse's income and assets are considered, and this can easily lead to ineligibility.

If both members of the couple are disabled, there are ramifications—asset limits are different for individuals and couples. The amount of assets a married couple is allowed to have and be eligible for SSI is $3,000. Every single person can have up to $2000 in assets.

Not only could one person lose their benefits, but both people can be denied for having the same exact amount of assets they had prior to marriage.

The simple act of sharing a bank account can make a person on SSI ineligible due to asset limitations, as the entirety of the bank account is considered for each person during their eligibility determination.

To make matters worse, SSI has a rule that people "living as married" are subject to these rules, without a full explanation of the definition of "living as married" so folks on SSI have to worry and wonder what will happen if they are in a committed relationship, even if they don't get a marriage license.

To protect yourself if you are in a relationship, be sure to separate your finances as much as possible, with separate bank accounts, and have proof you split your bills relatively evenly, as you would with a housemate, as opposed to a life partner.

I really feel for the folks on SSI who are worried about the marriage penalty, as it has the potential to destroy their lives—since most people on SSI are struggling to survive on that small amount of income and are forced to stay low-income in order to continue to get that financial support. The only way a married person can maintain SSI benefits if their income or assets are higher than the magic numbers are if they have their excess in an ABLE account (discussed in detail in **Navigating Disability Finances**) or can reliably and consistently prove they live separately, making up two separate households. This, for obvious reasons, is not an ideal situation for most people.

SSI eligibility may impact food stamps, income, and, most importantly, Medicaid to manage healthcare. The safest thing to do if on SSI is to not get married. The better you can protect yourself from appearing to "live as married", the safer you are.

While bills have been introduced in both the House of Representatives and Senate to correct the marriage penalty and update the asset limits (SSI Savings Penalty Elimination Act), they have not yet been passed. If passed, the asset limit for single individuals would jump to $10,000 and $20,000 for a couple (basically an update based on inflation) and then inflation-based updates would be applied moving forward. So far, the bills have been introduced in 2022, 2023 and 2024 but haven't gotten out of committee. (Translation: they have stalled and don't have a great chance of passing.)

The financial cost of marriage on SSDI

SSDI is based on individual work history and has fewer asset-related limitations. If the only benefit you receive is SSDI, which provides Medicare coverage and a monthly check, marriage isn't financially impossible, but access to any of the financially-based programs (pretty much all other social welfare programs) may be more challenging.

You will need to provide information about both your and your spouse's assets for all future requests of any sort. While some programs discuss household values (which could affect you and your partner from the moment you live together), sometimes only individual assets are considered for support.

You can apply as an individual for support if you are unmarried, but if you are married, your spouse's assets are always considered. If for any reason your partner later needs assistance, they will have their application process potentially impeded by your benefits and assets. As I mentioned above, SSI and other programs will consider spousal assets.

As an example, I know somebody who is on SSI benefits and is married to a person on SSDI. Because they are married, she only remains eligible for SSI if they live separately and maintain separate households.

If she wanted to live with him, she would lose her Medicaid coverage, but their marriage would not make her automatically eligible for his Medicare.

For tax purposes, a single person only collecting SSDI doesn't need to pay taxes because that income is too low. Once married, that same amount of money is added to their spouse's income, which usually will push their total income over that line, and likely bring up the overall taxes owed significantly. This means most or all the person on SSDI's disability income would become taxable due to their marriage. Is it the end of the world? Absolutely not. But if you are struggling with survival due to low income, you don't want to do anything that will reduce it further, so it behooves you to be aware of these associated costs.

Laws on healthcare

If these programs only provided money, I would not be as concerned. However, currently, the United States is in a health-care crisis. SSDI provides Medicare coverage and SSI provides Medicaid coverage. Often these are the only health care coverage we receive.

Losing our benefits starts the clock on losing our healthcare (if it doesn't immediately end our eligibility). People with disabilities, by definition, are more apt to need health care than anybody else. We have medications and medical care needed to maintain our quality of life, and in many cases, simply to stay alive.

If our spouses have health care, by marrying we are eligible to join their plan (though many plans nowadays don't require marriage for that eligibility), but that often comes with increased financial costs and assumes the spouse has health care in the first place. This places those of us with disabilities in a place of dependency on our partners and their employers. The right to theoretically use a spouse's possible benefits is generally not as useful as having a source of health insurance that isn't dependent on anyone's employment status.

This means that getting married puts a large additional financial burden on our spouse, increases our dependency on them, and makes leaving the relationship even more challenging should that become necessary. Should our spouse die, we may be in an exceptionally vulnerable place both emotionally and financially at a time of severe, life-altering trauma, which is never a good combination.

For the people who need Medicaid to survive, the risk of losing health insurance is especially significant (we discuss these details in Volume II). Medicaid provides for a variety of services essential for the survival of many people with more severe physical disabilities. Home Health Aides and other home and community-based services frequently do not have matches in the private sector, and for people who need those types of services, losing that coverage could be dangerous or even fatal.

Laws on medical decisions

One of the rights that comes with a legally recognized marriage is legal recognition as next-of-kin to your spouse.

This is extremely important in the case of severe injury (which may cause a disability), as it is the next-of-kin who often makes health-related decisions if the person who sustained the injury is unable to make their own medical decisions. In the case of a chronic and worsening condition, there is a high risk of the disabled person being unable to make some decisions in an emergency.

When a person is unmarried, legally their next-of-kin tends to be their parents, sibling/s, or adult child/ren, unless they have a living will (dictating their desires) or have designated somebody to have durable power of attorney through the appropriate documentation.

This means for a person with a disability, the decision not to marry can have substantial ramifications, especially if the relationship between their partner and their family is challenging, or the family, partner, and disabled individual are in disagreement about the best course of treatment.

This challenge can be remedied with a living will (which specifically states what your desires are) or legally recognized statement of who has your durable medical power of attorney (ability to make decisions for you) if you are incapacitated (either temporarily or permanently).

The LGBT community is especially familiar with challenges like this, as historically same-sex partners have been more likely to be rejected by their partner's families or ignored by medical professionals. Historically, some same-sex partners were prevented from even visiting their partner in the hospital, due to "family only" visitation policies at some hospital ICUs.

Though same-sex marriage is now legally recognized throughout the country, the associated biases still increase the risks for same-sex couples of being disregarded or ignored during emergencies. This makes life for a same-sex couple where one or both of them has a disability especially challenging and makes having documentation of medical authority even more vital. While a partner of a different sex may be assumed to be the spouse, the biases that exist in our society today makes that considerably less likely to be the case with a same-sex couple.

Again, in the case of medical decisions, it is possible to protect yourself by creating a living will, securing a medical power of attorney, or similar documentation, but that is an extra step and extra work when a legally recognized marriage guarantees that responsibility, and does not require additional paperwork.

Why my partner and I aren't getting married

My partner, Al, and I have been together since 2010.

He proposed on Halloween of 2016 and I proudly wear my lovely engagement ring. It's not traditional, but I love it!

We hope to have a commitment ceremony sometime in the next few years—a small ceremony and a big party to celebrate our love and commitment to one another. However, we have no intention of getting legally married. We aren't going to do that paperwork.

Why not? Because it is a financial and health risk for the both of us. My SSDI benefits aren't at risk, but we want to maintain my options for additional assistance if I need it. For some time, for example, I was supported by the NJ Workability program, which allowed me to have Medicaid benefits while employed.

This cut down on my medical expenses, as Medicaid generally covers the remainder of medical costs (while Medicare covers 80%) and allowed me to be eligible for additional supports like a Home Health Aide (which I did need at one point).

I let my Medicaid lapse years ago (not interested in worrying about their clawbacks), and while I could argue my way back onto the Workability program, I decided not to.

If Al and I had been married, getting on the Workability program would have required jumping through additional hoops, and at the time would have made Al's work income a potential issue if he found a better paying job. The rules around Workability have changed now, with no limitation placed on income (though you do need to pay for Medicaid coverage once your income passes a certain point) or assets.

Since then, the tables have turned a few times. After Al shattered his acetabulum, he was unable to work for the better part of a year, and we had a period where we weren't sure if he'd be able to work at all.

He had a spotty work history prior to that, caused by events outside of his control, including the great recession in 2008 followed by a brain injury in 2012 that kept him unable to contemplate working for over a year.

Due to this, he was ineligible for SSDI, which requires full-time employment for 5 of the previous 10 years (he has more than enough points to be eligible for retirement benefits). His only recourse would have been to apply for SSI.

If we were married, my benefits and assets would make his eligibility for SSI impossible.

Fortunately, he did recover enough to return to work, though he was only up for working about 30 hours a week rather than the usual 40.

I'm developing my work into a business (this book is another step in that direction) and hope I can supplement my income and give us a better quality of life, with a dream of someday earning enough I can decide to stop collecting SSDI altogether.

While SSDI doesn't have asset limits and so is unaffected by whether Al and I get married, most disability support programs are asset- and resource-based social welfare programs.

Right now, I don't need those supports. However, part of how I get through any major medical expense is by doing it at the hospital and then applying for financial assistance (if you are interested in how, and haven't read it already, I discuss the process in detail in Chapter 5 of **Navigating Disability Finances**).

I only need to provide the hospital with my financial information because I am legally single—but if Al and I were married, or shared bank accounts, I would have a lot more paperwork to file for that financial aid, and I'd be less likely to get full support.

If I had a severe symptom shift and needed more help with the basics of life, Medicare doesn't pay for Home Health Aides, so I'd need to get back on Medicaid to get that help. It's much easier for me to get that support as a single woman than a married one—and a lot less paperwork to turn in.

My big concern now, however, is Al himself. I'm very proud of him for getting the job he did, and for being able to work as much as he does. However, I'm very aware he is dealing with chronic pain and an autoimmune condition. Losing his job in February was rough for us, and him getting severely ill immediately after didn't help. He remains at risk for complications or future accidents, and while he is looking for work, we simply don't know how long it will be until he can find something that will work with his needs. His only backup option is SSI, which is a path both of us hope he will not need to take.

If he is married to me, he is ineligible for SSI and getting onto Medicaid might be a struggle. If we aren't married, he's easily eligible for Medicaid, and it wouldn't be hard for him to prove financial eligibility for SSI if he became unable to work.

While we are living on a financial edge like this, I want to keep both of us safe, and we have more options if we don't get married. So that's the plan.

The cost of not getting married

Getting married is something expected in our society. Even with divorce being relatively acceptable, there's still this assumption and expectation of marriage.

"When are you getting married?" is such a common question, and it's expected and assumed that dating leads to marriage.

Our society assumes two people who are couple and intend to spend their lives together should get married. Al and I, as a male and female couple, are expected to marry. We've had a lot of people assume we're married and refer to us as husband and wife. We generally don't bother correcting them because we have that degree of commitment to one another.

While same-sex couples may have slightly less of that pressure, any couple runs the risk of the partner or partner's family thinking they may be less valued because the legal niceties have not been completed. Without legally marrying, our properties and money (such as they are) will not automatically be given to our partner. Instead, if there isn't a will or other legal documentation, our families will need to sort things out, which may leave our partners in uncomfortable positions.

For Al and I, the only big "loss" is that I don't officially have the title of "Aunt" to his niblings, and he doesn't officially have the title of "Uncle" to my niblings (though we are occasionally referred to that way anyway).

In some families, there's a strong value placed on marriage and weddings—and in some cultures, individuals aren't expected to leave the family home until they get married, so marriage is the final step into full adulthood. I know for some families, not getting married is labeled as "living in sin" and children born out of wedlock are labeled as illegitimate.

Most of society considers marriage a positive, a sign of success, an expected milestone, and something that comes with many benefits. Unfortunately, for too many disabled people, ableism and our current social structure has instead turned marriage into something many disabled folks are penalized for and provides a reason to strip us of benefits.

I hate that we are forced in this direction—because too many disabled folks need Home Health aides or impossibly expensive medication to survive. Adding the stress of being unmarried despite societal pressure and fearing some SSA employee is going to decide you are "living as married" and end your benefits, isn't good for anyone.

The expense of getting divorced

Another reason why Al and I aren't getting married is because I never want us to have to contemplate getting divorced, especially not for healthcare/disability reasons. Up to 85% of marriages with severely disabled children end in divorce, and a good number of inter-abled marriages (especially when one member becomes disabled after marriage) end in divorce. Divorces are difficult under the best of circumstances but divorcing while adjusting to a disability definitely doesn't qualify as ideal.

> **I remember when I worked for the Division of Disability Services and a woman called about trying to get Medicaid.**
>
> They held her as ineligible because her estranged husband was paying her $1,000/month in support, and to be eligible for Medicaid that year, her unearned income needed to be under $973.
>
> The only advice we could give was to ask her ex to pay her $972/month so she could get Medicaid coverage.

Many people have had divorce suggested as the solution to their or their children's health care issue. It's an uncomfortable decision to have to make and one that can have a variety of negative ramifications for the couples and their social networks.

A friend's mother is very slowly dying from medical complications.

She and her father are discussing having him divorce her mother so Medicaid becomes an option.

While her father has moved out and has a new partner, he's uncomfortable with the idea of publicly abandoning his wife through divorce even though she's no longer capable of taking care of herself or even expressing herself. At this point, he's paying for full-time caregiving for her and it's draining the family of resources.

It seems to me one of the best ways to avoid needing to divorce for these reasons is to not get married in the first place.

I know that right now, and in the immediate future, Al and I are doing all right. However, I know as I get older, the chance of additional health issues increases, and the overall stress to my body increases. This doesn't guarantee I'll need extra help, but it does increase that possibility.

When Al and I first started dating, our only disability-related concern was my health. Since then, however, he has been through a Traumatic Brain Injury (TBI), a shattered acetabulum, and has been diagnosed with autoimmune pernicious anemia. It seems somewhat common for people with an autoimmune condition to develop additional challenges, and osteoporosis (which is why his acetabulum broke) is usually a progressive condition (we were able to just barely get his situation downgraded to severe osteopenia, but I'm uncertain how long that will last).

Al is already in pain and has weak bones. While there are many things he can do to slow the progression, he cannot reverse either challenge. He may not be able to work as long as he otherwise would have, and that's a reality that we have accepted.

How our families have dealt with our decision not to marry

Our families understand why we aren't married.

My mother and I had discussed this when I went onto SSDI and how it was somewhat likely I simply wasn't going to be legally married to anybody, though I definitely could have a life partner.

When Al and I had been dating about a year and decided to move in together, we explained to his parents that because of how disability benefits worked, it wasn't a good idea for us to get married, ever. Al's uncle lives on SSI, so they understood some of the challenges.

One of the main reasons we want to have a commitment ceremony is to give the kids a day where I officially become "Aunt Alison" and Al becomes "Uncle Al." We'd like to celebrate our love and have our families and friends intermingle more.

We haven't yet, mainly for financial reasons. I feel so fortunate our families are so loving and accepting. There's never been a negative comment about us living together without being married, and both our families have accepted both of us as part of the family.

We've got that even though we don't have a piece of paper or a specific date of commitment. I know that for many others, this simply isn't the case, and I am so grateful for what I do have.

Looking into the future

> **I can't see getting legally married in my future at the moment.**
>
> Al and I have built a comfortable life for ourselves—we've adopted two cats and the four of us are happily cohabitating.
>
> I am building my business and hoping eventually I'll have a consistent and high enough income that I can safely earn my way off SSDI. We're happily committed to one another and a ceremony or piece of paper isn't going to change that.

The disability community faces challenges others don't, and I'm not just talking about rampant ableism. We have the very real limitations our conditions cause and earning income doesn't remove those limitations (though it does give us more options on how to cope).

I would love to be part of a world where my marital status doesn't threaten my ability to get the support I need to manage my condition. We all deserve to be treated better, and the current "marriage penalty" doesn't improve anybody's quality of life but instead punishes disabled folks and inter-abled couples for wanting to have the same privileges as the rest of society.

People on SSI shouldn't lose their benefits because they want to publicly acknowledge their love for one another. None of us should need to choose between expressing our love and our own survival.

KEY POINTS

- **Marriage** is a societal norm and expectation and is assumed to be a positive life milestone that improves your life and status in society. This isn't always the case, and disabled people are often penalized in various ways for marrying.
- **Supplemental Security Income (SSI)** benefits include penalties for "living as married" or marrying. These include a reduction in permitted assets for the couple (as opposed to two single people) from $2,000 individually to $3,000 for the couple and can result in both people losing essential benefits.
- **Social Security Disability Insurance** benefits do not have a marriage penalty, but a married couple is, by definition, a household. This can have negative impacts on taxes and the disabled person's eligibility for needs-based programs.
- Health insurance is directly attached to SSI and SSDI benefits, so losing benefits also means losing Medicaid and/or Medicare coverage. This unfairly places the burden of insurance costs on the spouse of the disabled person, whose needs are often prohibitively expensive.
- **Medical decisions** are made by the next-of-kin if the individual is unable to make them. A spouse is legally next-of-kin. If in a long-term committed relationship that does not include marriage, the disabled individual must create legal documents to determine who makes these decisions if they can't.
- **Not marrying** has social costs for any couple, including the risk of a partner or their family feeling devalued or deprioritized or society in general viewing them as uncommitted, immature, or otherwise painted as a failure.
- **Divorce** is also expensive and messy. An unmarried couple can create arguments showing they are two separate households if this is necessary for the disabled individual to get essential supports. A married couple would need to divorce in order for them to be eligible.

RESOURCES

Social Security Administration. n.d. "SSI Income Rules." **https://www.ssa.gov/ssi/text-income-ussi.htm**.

Kenneally, Tim. 2019. "Medical Divorce: The Grim Reality of Expensive Health Care Bills." Observer. **https://observer.com/2019/08/medical-divorce-grim-reality-expensive-health-care-bills/**.

Hayes, Alison. Thriving While Disabled. n.d. "The U.S. Healthcare System Is Broken." **https://thrivingwhiledisabled.com/the-us-healthcare-system-is-broken/**.

GovTrack.us. n.d. "H.R. 5408 — 118th Congress: SSI Savings Penalty Elimination Act." **https://www.govtrack.us/congress/bills/118/hr5408**.

U.S. Congress. n.d. "H.R.3824 — 117th Congress: Supplemental Security Income Restoration Act of 2021." **https://www.congress.gov/bill/117th-congress/house-bill/3824/text**.

Kagan, Julia. 2023. "Power of Attorney (POA): Meaning, Types, and How and Why to Set One Up." Investopedia. **https://www.investopedia.com/terms/p/powerofattorney.asp**.

Kagan, Julia. 2023. "Living Will: Definition, Purpose, and How to Make One." Investopedia. **https://www.investopedia.com/terms/l/livingwill.asp**.

Kagan, Julia. 2023. "What (and Who) Is Next of Kin, and Why Does It Matter?" Investopedia. **https://www.investopedia.com/terms/n/next-of-kin.asp**.

RESOURCES WEBPAGE » CHAPTER 14

CHAPTER 15

Children and Disability
Risks and rewards as a parent with a disability

I am going to start this chapter with a disclaimer: I am not personally experienced with this topic. I am aware of some resources that may be useful, and felt this book would be incomplete without discussing this. My personal experience is one of deciding not to take the path of having children, and of my own awareness of and conversations with friends about being a disabled child or parent. With that in mind, let's discuss major considerations related to being a disabled parent and touch on considerations around having a disabled child.

Having a child is expensive

When you choose to have (biologically or through adoption) a child, there will be additional expenses, since you are now responsible for another human being. That's a given. As a person with a disability, you will have fewer usable hours in the day than abled people, and children take a lot of time and energy. It's possible you may run the risk of passing on the condition you have to the next generation, if your condition is hereditary and your child biologically yours. It's often easier to adopt disabled children, as too many people view the disability as a good reason to reject a child.

While there are government support programs to help low-income families, they face the same types of issues I've discussed throughout this book: the programs are challenging to find, don't provide enough money, and the people who administer the programs are likely to be biased against you. If you are primarily supported by social welfare programs, just surviving can be financially difficult—and adding a child to the mix is going to cost much more than you'll have added to your accounts by increasing your household size.

If you are considering adoption, it may be more difficult for you to adopt, as you have a minority identity potentially being held against you as you participate in that process.

If you are part of the LGBT community, adoption is generally the most affordable option, but is likely to be an uphill battle, especially with at least two minority identities being held against you. Social pressure may not push you towards having a child, but should you decide to do so, you will either need to fight bias to adopt a child or pay extra money in order to create a child that may genetically be yours or your partner's.

Even if you are in a relatively good financial situation, most disabilities are accompanied by additional expenses, so your decision to have a child will leave you struggling more in terms of both money and energy than your abled peers.

Not having a child can also be costly

At the same time, there is social pressure to have children as the obvious next step all straight-passing couples must want to take after they get married. While "when are you having kids" isn't asked as often as "when are you getting married" or "what do you do for a living", it is commonly assumed that all abled (or abled-passing) male-female couples are planning to have at least one child.

Socially, ableism frequently leads to visibly disabled people being treated as if they were children, and so the idea of them having children of their own does not always go over well. If you and/or your partner are visibly disabled, people may assume that you cannot (or do not) have sex, or that you cannot have a child due to medical complications, or that caring for a partner with a disability is equivalent to having a child, or that it is too much work to have both a disabled partner and a child. All these assumptions can be hurtful and are sometimes emotionally debilitating.

While it is financially less expensive to not have a child, it can be more expensive socially and emotionally. Having a child is another social milestone, one most people grow up expecting to reach, and not doing so can be upsetting. You may miss out on social opportunities, feel distanced from your community, or go through some form of grieving process over the loss of opportunity to have and raise a child.

There is a descriptive term I will share here, "childless not by choice", which describes people who wanted to have a child, but circumstances outside of their control prevented it. In Resources, I'll share a link to further information about this experience and support spaces related to it.

Only you can and should decide whether to try to have a child

This can be a very sensitive subject, and I want to be very clear here, only you (and your partner if you have one) should decide whether you try to have a child. Whether you are looking to be pregnant, cause a pregnancy, or adopt, you, as the potential parent, should be the one deciding if you are going to do so.

Discussions with your doctor about the safety or possibility of pregnancy makes sense, as does planning financially if you can, but having a disability should not be the primary or sole reason you don't have a child.

You shouldn't feel you must have a child because society expects you to, or due to other outside pressures. As you would be the (or one of the) primary caregiver/s to this child, it only makes sense to have a child if you want to have both the pleasure and challenges of caring for another human being for the rest of your (or their) life. It's impossible to know exactly how that will feel until you're there, but only you should decide if that's a responsibility and risk you are willing to take.

As disabled people, we can do anything our body/mind limitations do not prevent, though often the cost of doing some things may be more than they are for our abled peers. It is much harder for us to do all the things we want to do, but we can achieve the things we value most by prioritizing them and finding or creating solutions to the problems facing us.

So, if one of your high priorities in life is to have a child (or children), I absolutely believe in your ability to do so. Whether you plan (or end up) doing it with a partner (or partners) or as a single parent, I believe in you and your love for your child/ren. I support your choice. Whatever challenges might be in your way, I believe in your ingenuity and ability to find the solutions you need.

> ### Why Al and I are childless and okay with it
>
> All of the expenses listed above were reasons why Al and I hesitated to have children.
>
> We have never been in a good financial situation, and Al had grown up relatively poor and has strong feelings about not creating that sort of situation for his own child/ren.
>
> I recognized with how unpredictable my FND is, the stress of pregnancy and then raising a child was likely to increase my symptoms, leaving me uncertain about both my ability to care for my potential child, and my ability to do anything more than care for any child I might have. The physical process of having sex is difficult for me, due to pelvic floor dysfunction triggered by my FND. All the medical diagnoses I have are not directly inheritable (they aren't genetic anomalies that can be identified), but many do have a genetic component to them. Al and I are both nearsighted with astigmatisms and have depressive tendences. FND, depression, anxiety, and migraines all have genetic components and so any child we had would have a greater than average chance of inheriting any or all of these issues.
>
> Al and I had both assumed we'd have children, eventually, but eventually has never happened for us. With the medical struggles he has had, each one left him less sure of both his ability to care for a child and his ability to work enough to support one. We have recognized over the years that we have enjoyed our childfree lifestyle and have found other outlets for the parental feelings we do have.

Family is very important to us, and we live in the same county as his parents, my mother and her husband, Al's sister and her family, and one of my sisters and her children. Between us, we have six nieces and nephews (or niblings, to use the gender-neutral term), all of whom are close enough for us to see and spend time with regularly. We have good relationships with both sets of parents, and we recently moved in with his parents. We focus on being a good aunt and uncle to the kids and enjoy time with them as we have the spoons, knowing we can return them to their parents when we need a break or have an emergency.

We decided that the pitter-patter of furry feet was enough for us and have had cats throughout our relationship. While we do not have children, we do have an emotional and financial commitment to two small lives we invest time, energy, love, and money on.

We took time after I had to have a cervical biopsy (which increases the risk of complications to pregnancies) to discuss our history of opportunities for pregnancy and how we felt about having (or not having) a child. It was not an easy conversation, and I grieved the dream of having a child of my own. But Al and I agreed there hadn't been a point in our relationship where we strongly felt we should try to get pregnant or have a child, and this was nobody's fault, and it wasn't something either of us resented.

If our lives drastically improve financially, we may consider adopting a child at some point in the future, but we have agreed that we are content as a childless couple with niblings and cats to spoil.

Raising children when disability is involved

If you have children, I want you to be aware of a few of the largest challenges and of the supports available. There are some out there, but like the other supports I've mentioned in the book, the themes of scarcity and ableism remain.

Structural ableism increases the odds of a few different challenges, whether it's you or your child/ren (or both) that have a disability. As we've mentioned a few times, accessibility in general can be challenging. Especially if you and your child are both managing disabilities, these accessibility challenges can be multiplied, as all too often it's assumed a disabled person will always have an abled person with them (since obviously—ableism says—we can't participate in society without an abled person).

The risk of outsiders assuming incompetence or inability is higher, so you may be at greater risk of having your parenting skills questioned (including the risk of being reported to Child Protective Services or having a judge give priority to a spouse in the case of a divorce) or being harassed by others in positions of (perceived) power. These biases are not legal and should not be given additional weight, but I'm trying to prepare you for the non-medical risks that may occur.

As discussed early in the book, bias against people with disabilities is very real, and while we are a recognized, legally protected, minority class, having these legal protections and being safe can be two very different things. Progress has been made, but ableism is still part of our cultural norms, so be prepared.

As a parent to a child with a disability, many of the rules I've discussed throughout the book may apply to your child and may help you prepare your child's financial future. Especially if you and your child are both disabled, or your child's disability is very severe (and therefore usually very expensive to manage), it's important to know what protections and support they are eligible for.

Children can be eligible for SSI coverage starting at birth. The rules are a bit different for a child (under 18) than for an adult (18 or over). The biggest difference in terms of financial eligibility is the asset and income limits. While, as an adult, your income and assets are the primary consideration, for children, their parent's assets and income are, since their parents are legally and financially responsible for their care.

The calculation process for this, referred to as "deeming", is a bit complicated and links to help you understand it can be found in the

Resource section. If you (the parent) are collecting SSI or other needs-based benefits, your child is categorically eligible for SSI benefits and deeming rules aren't a necessary calculation. The goal of deeming is to only provide benefits for (abled) parents who need financial support to care for their disabled children. As we've discussed previously, these rules are based on multiple flawed premises, so many people who would benefit from this support will not be eligible, but that is typical of all the programs discussed throughout the book.

You want to know your (and your child's) rights when it comes to disability and education (discussed in Chapter 13). Your school district is responsible for some of the testing and support for children with (or suspected of having) disabilities, especially ones that impact learning.

As a parent, if your child has a disability, you are going to want to do a deep dive into their rights and how to protect them (Chapter 13 gives some good starting points). You will want to be prepared to push for testing or support if it is not immediately offered by the school.

As with so many other things, accessibility is too often not treated as a priority, but rather as an extra, so especially in a low-income school district (which statistically we are more likely to live in), you may need to push hard to ensure that your child gets the support they are legally eligible for. See Chapter 13 for more details.

KEY POINTS

- **Having a child is expensive.** Creating or adopting a new human being is going to cost a lot more money than not doing so. It is a huge responsibility that lasts a lifetime. Disabled people are often poor, and poor people are living with minimal extra money to pay these expenses.

- **Not having a child is expensive.** Society expects (abled) male-female couples to have children. Often, you're not viewed as fully adult until you're a parent. You may have always assumed you'd be a parent.

- **Childless Not By Choice.** A description of people who did not become parents due to life situations they could not control. The movement recognizes the grief that can accompany this lack.

- **Ableism has a strong influence on how you are treated.** If you are a disabled parent, you have a higher risk of being accused of neglecting or abusing your child/ren (or losing custody in a divorce). If you are disabled, others may try to discourage you from having children in the first place. If your child is (also) disabled, it's going to be harder for them (and you) to participate in society. None of this is legal, but it's likely to happen.

- **Choice** is the key issue. If you want to have a child, I believe in your ability to make it happen and successfully raise that child or children. If you do not wish to have a child, I fully support that decision as well. Just make sure that it is your decision, not one forced on you by outside influences or pressures.

RESOURCES

Wong, Alice, ed. 2024. **Disability Intimacy: Essays on Love, Care, and Desire**. New York: Vintage Books. This contains a few excellent stories about disabled pregnancy, parenting, and childcare (it also contains other excellent stories of other types of intimacy)

Matheis, Dave, ed. 2021. **A Celebration of Family: Stories of Parents with Disabilities.** Louisville, KY: Advocado Press. This shares experiences of parents with disabilities (and reprints my blog post on marriage and disability)

Malm, Sarah. 2021. "Grieving While Chronically Ill and 'Childless Not By Choice.'" Thriving While Disabled. July 30, 2021. **https://thrivingwhiledisabled.com/grieving-childless-not-by-choice/**.

RESOURCES WEBPAGE » CHAPTER 15

SECTION 3

Creating a Better Future

CHAPTER 16

Disability Rights Advocacy
Creating a better future

Let's talk about what could help us and our society improve. Since ableism is the root of many of the challenges we face, one of the most important things to do is simply to help people recognize their bias against people with disabilities and break it down. We're already working on that process.

Every disabled person who goes out in public or speaks on social media is taking steps to break down the bias. Our advocacy work looks somewhat different from other minority identities, but we're still out there advocating for ourselves.

By being visible or coming out as disabled, we're helping to break down barriers, educate those around us, and take needed steps to normalize disabled people simply being part of our communities.

In this book, we've gone over many of the struggles we face as disabled people and the extra challenges we need to overcome just to be treated as fully human. So, what will help solve these challenges?

I've got a few ideas to share with you—in this and the following chapters!

Bias training and education

People are trained by society that disabled people are to be pitied, and it is inspirational if we succeed, even in basic things expected by all of society. These beliefs need to change, and while work has absolutely been done towards us being treated fairly and being viewed as fully human and deserving of equitable treatment, this ideal has not yet been reached. Historically, too little thought has been put into accessibility, especially accessibility considerations beyond the bare minimum required by law.

Even as the largest minority, we still are consistently othered by societal messaging. Many people with disabilities can't even comfortably identify as disabled because societal ableism makes that feel like such a terrible identity to take on (or they feel that their disability isn't severe enough to count). While some people with disabilities embrace the identity (at least eventually), many more fight against it.

Since the industrial revolution, employers have sought employees who will slot into their organization with minimal challenges. Hiring a diverse workforce means more effort and less conformity, which can lead to beautiful results, but the process is messier (at least initially) and more effort on the part of the employer. It's unsurprising that laws and education are necessary for the integration of a more diverse set of employees. While integrating most minority identities requires shifts in work culture, integrating employees with disabilities requires cultural shifts, changes in the physical environment, and often shifts in workflows and hiring processes. It's a lot to change, and much of it is not (and sometimes cannot) be mandated by law.

Bias training, increased familiarity with accessibility and universal design concepts (another priority I'll discuss further on), and simply realizing how many disabled people they already know are all powerful tools to help individuals become more aware and less judgmental. The disability community is far from alone in this, as members of greater society have not fully made that realization about women, people of color, members of the LGBTQ+ community, and many other historically marginalized identities. All of us with historically marginalized identities need to work together and lift one another up, rather than fighting one another for a piece of the pie.

Bias trainings have been slowly growing in acceptance, but are frequently too short, too infrequent, or neglect discussing disability as an identity that faces these biases. The Diversity, Equity, Inclusion, and Belonging (DEIB) movement in professional settings is very important, but even many of these programs do not have the knowledge, the training, or the will to discuss disability within this framework.

While employers sometimes invest in training and workforce development with the goal of making their workforce more diverse, they do not always carry through on these goals, or do not consider accessibility throughout their hiring process. Bias is real, and not only do too many organizations not even bother to work on correcting these issues, too many trainers and professionals in this field are not as prepared to fully process accessibility and ableism as they might think.

The Covid-19 pandemic really emphasized the severity of ableism in the US (and likely other countries). Too many doctors assume having a disability automatically means lower quality of life[50,] and so prioritized abled patients over patients with disabilities even when ventilators and other resources were not limited[51.]

Later in the pandemic, the CDC (Centers for Disease Control) celebrated that we'd reached a point where most of the people dying from Covid-19 had one or more comorbidities (which translates into having other health conditions, a.k.a. having a disability). The recent change to no longer requiring masks or isolation when diagnosed with Covid-19 (and worse, the states considering or passing mask bans) further indicates a disregard for the safety of people more likely to catch or have a severe reaction to Covid-19 (a.k.a. people with disabilities).

Covid-19 has been a mass disabling event[52,] with an estimated one in 10 infections leading to long Covid[53,] which is still being defined as a condition, but has potentially permanently disabling impacts.

---

50   STAT. 2021. "Large Majority of Doctors Hold Misconceptions About People with Disabilities, Survey Finds." STAT. February 1, 2021. **https://www.statnews.com/2021/02/01/large-majority-of-doctors-hold-misconceptions-about-people-with-disabilities-survey-finds/**.

51   Shapiro, Joseph. 2020. "Oregon Hospitals Didn't Have Shortages. So Why Were Disabled People Denied Care?" NPR, December 21, 2020. **https://www.npr.org/2020/12/21/946292119/oregon-hospitals-didnt-have-shortages-so-why-were-disabled-people-denied-care**.

52   Davis, Hannah E., Lisa McCorkell, Julia Moore Vogel, and Eric J. Topol. 2023. "Long COVID: Major Findings, Mechanisms and Recommendations." Nature Reviews Microbiology 21: 133–146. **https://doi.org/10.1038/s41579-022-00846-2**.

53   National Institutes of Health (NIH). 2023. "Large Study Provides Scientists with Deeper Insight into Long COVID Symptoms." NIH News Releases, May 25, 2023. **https://www.nih.gov/news-events/news-releases/large-study-provides-scientists-deeper-insight-into-long-covid-symptoms**

When I got Covid-19, my mental health became much more variable, with me dropping into states of anxiety or depression much more quickly than ever before and getting out of those states became a bit more mentally slippery. It hugely increased my FND symptoms, leaving me needing another round of intense physical therapy to regain my hard-won control over my body.

Too many people think Covid-19 is like a cold or flu, something that is survivable and generally leaves no long-term impact. While it may be true in some cases, people are much more likely to get long Covid than have long-term impacts from a flu virus or many other common viral infections.

All this leads back to my initial point: unless a person has actively educated themselves, most people have severe bias against people with disabilities, and even educators in the field of Diversity, Equity, Inclusion, and Belonging don't always recognize the practice of ableism.

RESOURCES

Pulrang, Andrew. 2021. "3 Mistakes to Avoid When Including Disability in Your DEI Programs." Forbes, August 27, 2021. **https://www.forbes.com/sites/andrewpulrang/2021/08/27/3-mistakes-to-avoid-when-including-disability-in-your-dei-programs/**.

Bucholtz, Sydney. 2022. "DEIB: Who Is Impacted & Why It's Important." InclusionHub, December 12, 2022. **https://www.inclusionhub.com/articles/why-deib-is-important**.

Demystifying Disability by Emily Ladau: "Ladau, Emily. 2021. Demystifying Disability: What to Know, What to Say, and How to Be an Ally. Emeryville: Ten Speed Press."

Zheng, Lily. n.d. Lily Zheng – DEI Strategist & Consultant. Accessed April 12, 2025. **https://www.lilyzheng.co/**. **LinkedIn+4Instagram+4Harvard Business Review+4**

RESOURCES WEBPAGE » CHAPTER 16

CHAPTER 17

Enforcing the ADA

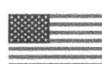 **UNITED STATES OF AMERICA**

Enforcing ADA Laws

Enforcement of the laws already in place and prioritizing the maintenance of accessibility tools could make a huge difference. Shifting expectations from disabled people being responsible for reporting accessibility failures to proactively confirming spaces, events, and processes are accessible could be a huge victory for the disability community.

As it stands, the laws on the books related to disability are decent, though there is always room for improvement. However, these laws have no teeth behind them, as minimal, if any, effort is put into enforcing them. Currently, enforcement of ADA laws falls squarely on the shoulders of people with disabilities, as we are expected to sue those who fail to follow these laws for their failure to do so[54].

Doctor's offices should all have ways to weigh patients who are full-time wheelchair users, and wheelchair users should get full bodied exams on the examining tables. Does your doctor's office have that ability? Most, if not all, of mine don't.

---

54 U.S. Department of Justice. n.d. "Cases." ADA.gov. Accessed April 12, 2025. https://www.ada.gov/cases/.

Public transportation has laws about accessibility, and while the work has been done to make the vehicles accessible (kneeling buses, wheelchair lifts or ramps, speaker systems for announcements, light boards in the front of the bus or train car to indicate the next stop), the work of maintaining those features seems to be very low priority. It shouldn't be.

If airports were immediately held responsible for the full cost of repairing the specialized wheelchairs they damaged (or if wheelchair users were able to use their chairs on the flight through use of tie downs or similar tools), I think (and hope) wheelchairs and wheelchair users would be treated much better by airlines.

We all deserve to be treated equitably and with respect. Simply enforcing the laws already on the books when it comes to disabilities and accessibility tools would make a huge difference in today's society.

All it takes is the will and better distribution of funds. Unfortunately, both ableism and classism make this more difficult. Many laws that protect us exist. Too many of them are unenforced and therefore ignored.

An outside regulatory agency that can fine, unendorse, or otherwise penalize organizations that fail to maintain accessibility standards could really help improve accessibility for the disability community.

As things stand, even members of the disability community cannot proactively fight for our rights, but instead one of us must first be directly damaged by an organization's failure to comply with the ADA[55]. As I discussed back in Chapter 4, classism has a huge influence on the law itself, specifically by making the legal process easier if you have more money to throw at the problem. Since disabled people are disproportionately poor, it only makes sense to help nullify this issue by financially backing other parts of the government to improve compliance with the law.

Officials tasked with inspection and enforcement (as exist with many other types of safety regulations), would likely improve compliance to ADA regulations.

---

55 Williams, Pete. 2023. "Disability Rights Activist Faces Supreme Court Showdown over Hotel Accessibility." NBC News, October 4, 2023. **https://www.nbcnews.com/politics/supreme-court/disability-rights-activist-faces-supreme-court-showdown-hotel-accessib-rcna76512**.

CHAPTER 18

Reframing Ableism and Working to be Anti-Ableist

Work has already been done by many civil rights leaders and disability justice advocates to allow all people equal rights. Laws have already been passed to help level the playing field.

But enforcement of the laws is lacking. Laws on the books aren't necessarily followed if nobody enforces them. We've seen too much proof unregulated or under-regulated industries tend to take shortcuts when it comes to following the rules.

As we've discussed throughout this book, ableism and bias against disability is deeply rooted in our legal, social, and welfare systems. Removing the ableism isn't easy, because it's baked into most laws and regulations.

Pulling back to the parallels I see between ableism and racism, so much of this is about changing people's perspective. Ibram X. Kendi's book on being an anti-racist rings incredibly true to me, and I can see that similar beliefs about disability are appropriate. It isn't enough to individually not be racist or not be ableist, because the system itself already has these traits built into it.

To truly protect and support people with marginalized identities, we need to recognize the bias in the laws, structures, and institutions themselves and change them to remove the bias. We don't just need to not be ableist, we need to be actively anti-ableist to truly have a good chance of being treated equally.

It isn't enough to recognize wheelchair users aren't confined to their chairs but freed by them. We have to work to remove the social, legal and architectural barriers that make it harder for people with disabilities to fully participate in society. This means the barriers need to be recognized, the bias needs to be measured, and the laws need to be changed so they are enforced, including having penalties that are more, not less, expensive than the cost of complying.

There should be curb cuts on every sidewalk, ramps instead of (or alongside) stairs, and every building, public or private, should be physically accessible. All crosswalks should have sound indicators as well as the visual ones we are used to. Part of maintenance of all public transportation should include ensuring the vehicle is fully accessible, and the repair of accessibility tools should be as important as other forms of maintenance. Wouldn't the world be a better place if events had quiet spaces to rest in, if captions came standard on everything, doors were always easy to open, and everything was designed with accessibility in mind?

Currently accessibility tools are frequently treated as extras, rewards, and add-ons. They're something the company will consider later or might add to the existing structure after the fact. Too often, "later" never happens. As things stand, accessibility is a legal requirement, and not part of the initial plan. Like other forms of legal compliance, accessibility is often considered last, rather than first, making it feel burdensome to abled folks and reinforcing the idea of accessibility as a form of appeasement to special interests. There is an alternative perspective to this too: the concept of universal design, which centers the goal on being useful for all people, rather than the average person.

RESOURCES

Kendi, Ibram X. 2019. **How to Be an Antiracist**. New York: One World.

Yu, Tiffany. 2024. **The Anti-Ableist Manifesto: Smashing Stereotypes, Forging Change, and Building a Disability-Inclusive World**. New York: Hachette Go.

RESOURCES WEBPAGE » CHAPTER 18

CHAPTER 19

Embracing Universal Design

Unsurprisingly, universal design was created by a person with a disability. Ronald Mace, one of many people impacted by polio, became a full-time wheelchair user by the age of 10. He defined universal design as **"design that's usable by all people, to the greatest extent possible, without the need for adaptation or specialized design."**

> 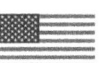 **UNITED STATES OF AMERICA**
>
> Currently, the ADA has requirements for buildings in the US to follow "Accessible Design" standards, which were created in 1991 and revised in 2010. The goal of accessible design is for the subject to be accessible for people with a (specific) disability, whether or not it is accessible for everyone. This means that accessible design focuses on following the law, and generally on the needs of a specific portion of the disability community (such as wheelchair users), rather than the community as a whole.

While having things designed specifically so that wheelchair users, people who are blind or low-vision, and d/Deaf people (for example) can use them is helpful, it reinforces the "othering" of the community and may fail to support multiply-disabled individuals (such as those who are deaf-blind, or wheelchair users with Autism Spectrum Disorder). This process reinforces the societal perspective of doing "extra" things for the disability community, as well as reinforcing segregation-style ideas of separate but equal resources (for example, compare the image of two water fountains side-by-side at different heights to the image of two water fountains side-by-side with race-based labels).

In contrast, universal design principles focus on creating spaces usable for all people, which includes, but is not limited to, people with disabilities. This means that ramps and elevators are part of the design process, rather than afterthoughts. But there's much more to it than that—universal design is about ensuring necessary information is communicated clearly (whatever is happening in the space and regardless of the sensory limitations of the user), can be accessed and used by any person (regardless their body size, mobility, or posture) and accommodate different preferences and abilities. With universal design, some assistive technologies may be unnecessary, but spaces using universal design principles should work with assistive technologies as appropriate. The point of universal design is to make the space accessible and usable for everyone, rather than only abled or disabled people.

There are **seven principles of universal design**. The first is to **create spaces that are of equitable use** (helpful for people with diverse abilities or needs). Secondly, the **space must have flexibility of use** (accommodate a range of individual preferences and abilities). It needs to be **simple and intuitive to use** (no matter what the user's prior experiences, knowledge level, language skills, or concentration level may be). **Spaces must provide perceptible information** (no matter what is happening in the environment or what the user's sensory limitations may be). **The spaces must have a high tolerance for error** (minimized risk of injury if something is used improperly) and **require little physical effort** (it should take minimal strength or dexterity). The final principle is that **the size of and space around everything involved should allow ease of use for any individual, regardless of their size, posture, or mobility** (no matter if the person is, for example, a Little Person, a wheelchair user, or tall with full mobility).

In the Resources section, you'll see links to several sites that discuss universal design, including many examples of universal design in architecture. The parks, public spaces, buildings, and more designed using universal design principles can be beautiful and functional for all people, rather than just a majority. Again, universal design isn't focused on disabilities but works to ensure that people with disabilities are included in all considerations from the beginning of the project.

While universal design was originally an architectural concept, its usage has expanded into many fields and disciplines. This includes work done in internet technology (the World Wide Web Consortium (W3C) created the Web Content Advisory Guide (WCAG) to ensure accessibility for all), education (discussed below), product creation (following the same principles as architecture), and much more.

Websites are expected to be WCAG compliant (often this is a stated prerequisite for site designers), but too many people don't fully understand what that means or why it's expected. The idea of adopting a set of rules intended to provide equal access for all to all websites would be incredibly helpful, and while many websites are fully accessible and often fit universal design principles, there are many that are not and do not. The point of the WCAG principles is to make all websites perceivable, operable, understandable, and robust. This translates into full accessibility whether you can see, hear, use a mouse, or have a learning disability or other condition or minority identity.

Universal Design in Education (UDE) is discussed in detail by Dr. Sheryl Bergstahler (her paper is linked in the resources section), as the combination of universal design in architecture (making places of learning accessible for all students), WCAG compliance (making sure all technologies used by educators are perceivable, operable, understandable, and robust), and UDL principles, discussed below.

Universal Design for Learning (UDL) is an underused yet vital tool for educators. UDL recognizes children learn best in different ways at different rates, and different tools help different students more than others.

Like architectural universal design, UDL focuses on inclusion and belonging. Instead of teaching one way and expecting all students to adapt (our modern system, with legal requirements to include children with disabilities), UDL recognizes students learn differently from one another, and provides information in a variety of ways so all students have an equal opportunity to succeed.

Flexibility in teaching and testing methods can allow all students opportunities to better absorb and retain information, including students with learning disabilities or other conditions that impact their ability to collect, process, or express information.

The philosophy behind all forms of universal design is not antagonistic to accessibility, but inclusive of it. Modern society is still focused on normative expectations. Things are (and have been for the past couple of hundred years) designed primarily by and for the "average" person (which somehow is always a straight, white, cis, abled, younger man). By shifting our focus as a society from conforming to normative expectations to celebrating diversity of experiences, we can create a better world for all of us.

RESOURCES

Universal Design Project. n.d. "Definition of Universal Design." Accessed April 12, 2025. **https://universaldesign.org/definition**.

Universal Design Institute. n.d. Universal Design Institute. Accessed April 12, 2025. **https://www.udinstitute.org/**.

U.S. Department of Justice. n.d. "2010 ADA Standards for Accessible Design." ADA.gov. Accessed April 12, 2025. **https://www.ada.gov/law-and-regs/design-standards/**.

Universal Design Project. n.d. "Accessible vs. Universal Design." Accessed April 12, 2025. **https://universaldesign.org/accessible-vs-universal-design**.

ArchDaily. n.d. "Universal Design." Accessed April 12, 2025. **https://www.archdaily.com/tag/universal-design**.

Re-thinking The Future. n.d. "Inclusive Spaces: Implementing Universal Design Principles in Urban Architecture." Accessed April 12, 2025. **https://www.re-thinkingthefuture.com/architectural-community/a12838-inclusive-spaces-implementing-universal-design-principles-in-urban-architecture/**.

World Wide Web Consortium (W3C). n.d. "Web Content Accessibility Guidelines (WCAG) Overview." W3C Web Accessibility Initiative (WAI). Accessed April 12, 2025. **https://www.w3.org/WAI/standards-guidelines/wcag/**.

U.S. Department of Justice. n.d. "Guidance on Web Accessibility and the ADA." ADA.gov. Accessed April 12, 2025. **https://www.ada.gov/resources/web-guidance/**.

Burgstahler, Sheryl. n.d. "Universal Design in Education: Principles and Applications." DO-IT Center, University of Washington. Accessed April 12, 2025. **https://www.washington.edu/doit/universal-design-education-principles-and-applications**.

Understood. n.d. "What Is Universal Design for Learning (UDL)?" Accessed April 12, 2025. **https://www.understood.org/en/articles/universal-design-for-learning-what-it-is-and-how-it-works**.

RESOURCES WEBPAGE » CHAPTER 19

CHAPTER 20

Universal Benefits

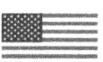 **UNITED STATES OF AMERICA**

If the US adopts universal healthcare, one of the big hurdles for the disability community in terms of both marriage and employment will go down, which would be wonderful.

As things stand, all disabled people are hampered by health insurance concerns.

For disabled people who are able to work full-time, their employer's healthcare plan is a major stressor. They need to maintain employment and generally get a more expensive healthcare plan and still pay more than the average person in out-of-pocket healthcare expenses.

For those of us who are not able to work full–time, we either are on disability-based programs like SSI or SSDI and worried about whether we can afford to earn our way off the programs (or so scared of that happening we don't try to work at all), or folks are earning their way off of benefits and then worrying about how they will get healthcare coverage.

With the habit Social Security has had lately of clawing back benefits (discussed in detail in Volume II), too many disabled folks and retirees are finding themselves in the untenable position of owing Social Security money with no way to repay the debt and often being denied benefits for months.

Having the US adopt a single-payer program, such as a form of Medicare for All[56,] would mean employment and health insurance are permanently separated from one another.

By doing that, most people with disabilities (and most poor people in general) would have a huge stress lifted from them.

We all would be able to get the medical care we needed, and the overall cost of the care would be reduced.

Would there be new problems or challenges? Of course—but it would be a challenge we were all facing together as a society rather than having us fractured into tiny struggling communities. It is a global challenge, and many other countries have already found some partial solutions—as I've discussed in many of the international sections of various chapters in both this book and the next.

Currently, health insurance providers try not to cover disabled folks, and make the process of getting care obscenely expensive. With single-payer coverage, the cost of medications and treatment would decrease dramatically, and the entire healthcare industry would become simpler, more streamlined, and be much easier for everyone to understand and use.

The combination of separating health insurance from employment and reducing healthcare costs would make a huge difference in both our quality of life as disabled people and our ability to work and earn money.

Current systems in other countries with single payer healthcare do have their own issues and challenges, as well as gaps in coverage for people with disabilities that each country handles in its own unique way (I give multiple examples in Volume II).

---

56 Booth, Stephanie. 2020. "Medicare for All: What Is It and How Will It Work?" Healthline, August 26, 2020. **https://www.healthline.com/health/what-medicare-for-all-would-look-like-in-america**.

> I would love it if the single-payer program the US eventually takes these challenges into account and creates a single plan that covers all individuals, and which is designed with a focus on handling the needs of people with disabilities, rather than the average (white, straight, abled, male) person. Will that happen? It's unlikely to happen anytime soon, but it is a goal to strive for—and learning more about the costs and benefits of plans enacted in other countries can definitely help us create something even better.

Let's Talk About Universal Basic Income

The other major change that would really help the disability community would be creating **universal basic income** (UBI) or developing another financial support system that doesn't have financial requirements tied in with disability supports.

As things stand, for disabled people to get any kind of help, we need to be poor, and that isn't fair for anybody.

What do I mean? Well, as we've discussed in this book, the current system effectively punishes you for trying to succeed. If you earn a dollar over any program's limits, you often lose up to hundreds or thousands of dollars of support.

The fear and anxiety around losing needed support for just a small amount of additional earnings (especially when the rules are so confusing, convoluted, and subject to interpretation) means it's emotionally and intellectually taxing to even consider earning your way off your support programs.

Even if you decide it's worth the effort, you now have many calculations to make to ensure you thread the needle of staying under the various earning amounts and to carefully document your process and health until or unless you can sustainably triple or quadruple your income over a relatively short period of time.

The struggle it took to get the benefits in the first place takes a toll on you and increases your desire to never go through those dehumanizing processes again, increasing your stress, which can increase the likelihood of you experiencing some form of relapse or symptom increase.

From a government structural perspective, there are a huge number of people maintaining and running all the social welfare and social security programs. The rules are complicated, checking compliance takes resources, and paperwork takes time.

If we dismantled all those systems, it's quite possible those cost savings would end up being similar to the expense of running a reasonable UBI program. Since that would be a monthly check or direct deposit to everyone, it would require minimal oversight and no means testing (the process of determining if the individual is still poor enough for benefits).

When the Covid-19 stimulus checks went out, one of the issues was the checks were all means-tested, so wealthier people didn't get a check. The time and effort spent on means testing every citizen for eligibility cost more than sending everyone a check. And if everyone gets the money, wealthier people are less likely to complain about the process.

Having UBI would protect us from much of the trauma and ableism we currently are subjected to. So much of the application process for benefits is about detailing social failures, and it is a shameful experience for the applicant, worsening mental health and self-belief at a time when they are already vulnerable.

If instead, we always have some money coming in, and working gives us additional money without the additional stresses, each person will work the amount that they feel able to do and take time off when needed.

By combining UBI and Universal Health Care, those of us living with disabilities will face considerably less financial stigma and stress and be better able to take care of ourselves and heal or learn to manage our conditions more quickly.

RESOURCES

Universal Health Care

U.S. News & World Report. n.d. "The Case for Universal Health Care." U.S. News & World Report. Accessed April 12, 2025. https://health.usnews.com/health-care/for-better/articles/the-case-for-universal-health-care.

Zieff, Gabriel, Zachary Y. Kerr, Justin B. Moore, and Lee Stoner. 2020. "Universal Healthcare in the United States of America: A Healthy Debate." Medicina 56 (11): 580. https://doi.org/10.3390/medicina56110580

Universal Basic Income

Investopedia. n.d. "What Is Universal Basic Income (UBI), and How Does It Work?" Accessed April 12, 2025. https://www.investopedia.com/terms/b/basic-income.asp.

International Monetary Fund (IMF). 2018. "What Is Universal Basic Income?" Finance & Development, December 2018. https://www.imf.org/en/Publications/fandd/issues/2018/12/what-is-universal-basic-income-basics.

Stanford Basic Income Lab. n.d. "What Is UBI?" Accessed April 12, 2025. https://basicincome.stanford.edu/about/what-is-ubi/.

Forbes Advisor. n.d. "Universal Basic Income Programs." Accessed April 12, 2025. https://www.forbes.com/advisor/personal-finance/universal-basic-income-programs/.

RESOURCES WEBPAGE » CHAPTER 20

CHAPTER 21

Thriving With Your Disability IS Advocacy
What can you do right now?

You can live out loud. Simply by going outside and interacting with people, folks with apparent disabilities are doing work to break down the stigma and helping shake loose some of the bias we all face.

For folks like me, whose disabilities are not easily apparent, asking for accommodations when needed and being transparent about having a disability can be a game-changer.

Our whole society has an ableist and classist bent. It's obvious in the way our social welfare programs are organized, and in the structure of our social security system and the tools we have to help disabled folks survive. That does not mean it needs to stay that way, or that we can't improve the situation.

Simply by participating in society, we are taking steps towards disability equity. By pointing out the inequality and bias, we get people thinking about their complicity in structural ableism. Education is a huge and vital part of this process as too many people simply don't think about ableism since it's so ingrained in society. We all deserve to be treated equitably.

Keep up with disability-related news and actions. I've shared many resources throughout this book and the next that should help you know what's going on, from a legal and financial perspective, with disability rights and support programs for disabled people.

Stay curious as you have the energy, and support social campaigns designed to protect or expand our rights. I recommend following the AAPD (American Association of People with Disabilities) as they often organize events and actions surrounding disability rights. I know your life already has challenges, and you're already facing an uphill battle. I need you to take care of yourself first.

Make sure you have food, shelter, space to think, and the other necessities of life. Be sure to give yourself a purpose. But once you've done that, remember all the other disabled folks who are still struggling for these things. Whatever work we do towards disability equity should help other disabled folks have an easier time taking those steps in the future.

RESOURCES

Organizations and Projects

United Nations. 2018. Disability and Development Report. New York: United Nations. **https://www.un.org/development/desa/disabilities/publications/disability-and-development-report.html**.

Autistic Self Advocacy Network (ASAN). n.d. Autistic Self Advocacy Network. Accessed April 12, 2025. **https://autisticadvocacy.org**.

International Disability Alliance (IDA). n.d. International Disability Alliance. Accessed April 12, 2025. **https://www.internationaldisabilityalliance.org/**.

Disability Rights International (DRI). n.d. Disability Rights International. Accessed April 12, 2025. **https://www.driadvocacy.org/**.

World Institute on Disability (WID). n.d. World Institute on Disability. Accessed April 12, 2025. **https://wid.org/**.

Disability Council International (DisabCouncil). n.d. Disability Council International. Accessed April 12, 2025. **https://disabilitycouncilinternational.org/**

Disability Visibility Project. n.d. Accessed April 12, 2025. **https://disabilityvisibilityproject.com/**

American Association of People with Disabilities (AAPD). n.d. "Home." Accessed April 12, 2025. **https://www.aapd.com/**.

Sins Invalid. n.d. Sins Invalid. Accessed April 12, 2025. **https://www.sinsinvalid.org**.

The Kelsey. n.d. The Kelsey. Accessed April 12, 2025. **https://thekelsey.org**.

HEARD (Helping Educate to Advance the Rights of the Deaf). n.d. HEARD. Accessed April 12, 2025. **https://www.heardproject.org**.

Individuals and Blogs

Abayomi-Paul, Tinu. 2024. "Honoring the Life and Legacy of Tinu Abayomi-Paul." Calling Up Justice, October 20, 2024. **https://callingupjustice.com/honoring-the-life-and-legacy-of-tinu-abayomi-paul/**.

Barbarin, Imani. n.d. Crutches and Spice. Accessed April 12, 2025. **https://crutchesandspice.com/**.

Pulrang, Andrew. n.d. Andrew Pulrang – Disability and Media Contributor. Accessed April 12, 2025. **https://www.forbes.com/sites/andrewpulrang/**.

Piepzna-Samarasinha, Leah Lakshmi. 2018. **Care Work: Dreaming Disability Justice**. Chicago: Aquarius Press.

Clare, Eli. 1999. **Exile and Pride: Disability, Queerness, and Liberation**. Cambridge, MA: South End Press.

Wong, Alice. 2020. **Disability Visibility: First-Person Stories from the Twenty-First Century.** New York: Vintage Books. (and several more)

Girma, Haben. 2019. **Haben: The Deafblind Woman Who Conquered Harvard Law.** New York: Twelve Books.

Thompson, Vilissa. n.d. VilissaThompson.com. Accessed April 12, 2025. **https://www.vilissathompson.com**.

Hashtag Activism

#CripTheVote. n.d. #CripTheVote Blog. Accessed April 12, 2025. **https://cripthevote.blogspot.com/**.

#BlackDisabledLivesMatter and #DisabilityTooWhite – Launched by Vilissa Thompson,

#NothingAboutUsWithoutUs – Essential framing for inclusive policymaking and discourse.

21 » Thriving With Your Disability IS Advocacy **» 249**

RESOURCES WEBPAGE » CHAPTER 21

Closing Letter

Thank you so much for joining me on this journey! I have loved the process of writing and editing this book, and I hope you've found it useful and helpful on your journey through disability. There's so much I've wanted to share, and it feels so good to put it out for you to read!

It has been quite a journey. The initial concept for this series was an outline for an online course, which I was tentatively calling "Survivor's Guide to Disability Finances". The course has yet to be created, but multiple people I shared the idea with immediately responded with "Alison, that's a BOOK." So, I decided to make that happen. After many conversations with various people, I eventually decided to self-publish with 3 ferns publishing...but then got pulled into an almost year-long misadventure with a different publishing company who let me down. I returned to 3 ferns, and I'm so grateful to Leesa Ellis, the owner of 3 ferns, for all the support she has lavished on me and these books! Initially, they were intended to be a single book (**Thriving While Disabled: Navigating Disability Finances**), but I discovered that my wordcount was too high to easily be a single book. Thank you, Leesa, for suggesting this solution, and for handling all the necessary adjustments to make this possible!

In the meantime, as I allude to throughout the books, my life was full of changes. Between the day I decided to make the book happen, and the day I'm writing this missive, I've experienced more life upsets than I had in most of the last 5 or 6 years, if not longer. Al's employer went out of business in February 2023, which impacted our finances and Al's healthcare (we still haven't been reimbursed for March's COBRA payment!).

Al's been through another major medical scare, though at least this time (thankfully) there doesn't appear to be any permanent damage. Al and I lost our apartment and are now in a very different living situation, having moved ourselves and our cats in with his parents (the process started in mid-October and finally finished December 20th, 2024). Things have been unpredictable here, with his father dealing with a heart attack in July 2024, a second heart surgery just before Thanksgiving, and a stroke in January! I'm grateful we've moved in and are able to support his parents through it, and that they were happy to open their home to us.

We've been getting extra time in with my sister and her children the past few years, which has been wonderful. I'm very proud of her, and while sometimes tiring, I'm so grateful to get to spend more time with her and my niblings than I could earlier in their lives.

I was inspired by the 2024 election results to adjust the book to bring in more information about how other countries handle healthcare, disabilities and related topics. On that front, I'm so grateful to all the people who helped me gain more information and wider perspectives: Em, Robert, Stephanie, Mericel, Lara, Frederick, and many others who shared little factoids, stories, and bits of experience that may have made it into the book. I want to thank Carrie Kellenburger for looking this book over, giving advice on publishing processes and generally inspiring me with her awesomeness and enthusiasm. I want to thank Sheryl Chan for long ago planting the knowledge in my mind that the disability experience is pretty universal, which is what allowed me to pivot the book as rapidly as I did.

I have many family members, friends and acquaintances who shared stories that inspired me, got me thinking, or were mentioned in the book, including Mike, Vera, Kari, Amanda, Emily, Lindsey, Mom, Milton and Stuart, and so many more! I'm so grateful for your stories, experiences, trust, and love.

An extra shout-out to Mary Ann Hill, who excitedly took on developmental and copy editing these books at the last minute, after I realized my manuscript was so much longer than expected. She dived in with a will and excitement, sharing that deadlines help her focus. I am so grateful for her help.

I hope that you found these stories and experiences useful and that they helped you see just how connected we all are. Having a disability is tough, and living in an ableist world makes it tougher. We all deserve to thrive, and I hope this book has helped you get closer to that ideal!

Thank you,

Alison

Next Steps With Alison!

I'm so glad you've kept reading! I've created multiple online courses and talks that you may be interested in, most of which play on similar themes to what I've discussed in the books.

thrivingwhiledisabled.com/my-programs

If you have decided to apply for disability benefits, I'm here to guide you through:

thrivingwhiledisabled.com/applying-for-disability-coaching

If you are on benefits and contemplating work, but want support for that process:

thrivingwhiledisabled.com/working-and-self-employment-on-disability-coaching

In the meantime, please join my email list, and keep up with all I have to offer! I anticipate creating a new program to help folks keep getting one step closer to thriving, once I recover from the initial marketing of these books (and maybe give myself a month or two off).

About the Author

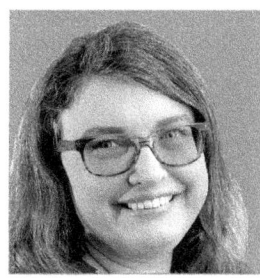

Alison Hayes is the founder and driving force behind her coaching business, Thriving While Disabled. This book has evolved from her blog. Her business has expanded to encompass coaching, training, and educational materials that help people with disabilities navigate the many broken systems which make their lives difficult.

The goal of her business is to empower her fellow disabled folks to know and protect their rights, recognize their worthiness as human beings, and find their own path to purpose.

Her wish is that you can thrive while managing society's perception and treatment of you as a person with a disability!

Alison and her partner Al live in New Jersey with their cats (one of whom is also chronically ill) and enjoy watching horror movies together. She's also a big reader of science fiction and fantasy books.

APPENDIX

Glossary

Glossary

ABLE Account – Achieving a Better Life Experience Account – A form of savings program specifically for people with disabilities who became disabled before the age of 26 (On January 1, 2026, the age will be raised to 46). Money in this account is not considered for any government benefits program and the money in the account can only be used for disability-related expenses (including housing and food).

Abled – Any person who is neurotypical and has no mental or physical handicaps or bodily differences outside of socially acceptable normative standards. Opposite of disabled.

Ableism – The view that disabled people are less human/worthy of respect due to having disabilities. The concept parallels sexism, racism, etc. except the bias is specifically against actual or perceived disabilities.

ACA – Affordable Care Act – Formally known as the Patient Protection and Affordable Care Act (PPACA), and informally referred to as "Obamacare", this comprehensive healthcare reform law was enacted March 2010. The primary goals were to expand Medicaid coverage to all people with income below 138% of the FPL (at time of writing, only 10 states have not expanded coverage), make healthcare plans more affordable to people with income up to 400% of the FPL, and support innovations to medical care delivery methods that generally lower the cost of healthcare. Another powerful component of this law was the closing of the "pre-existing condition" clause in health insurance.

ACA Marketplace – Website showcasing health insurance plans available for purchase. Sponsored by the federal government, many of these plans are available at a much lower rate due to a combination of tax breaks and government underwriting. These plans are generally available at those reduced costs for people whose incomes are up to 400% of the FPL, and intended primarily for individuals and families whose employers do not provide health insurance. Some states have their own ACA Marketplaces, while many utilize the federal site. These insurance plans are available during the Open Enrollment Period, and for people experiencing a Qualifying Life Event.

Accessible – Something designed to be easily entered, understood, or appreciated. Used by the disability community to indicate that something can be used regardless of ability. "Accessible" has been adopted by much of the disability community to replace the term "handicapped". Examples: "Accessible parking has the blue lines and wheelchair user icon." "I wanted to read up on that political candidate, but their site wasn't accessible for my screen reader." "Is this space scent-free, or is it inaccessible to people with chemical sensitivities?"

ACL – Administration for Community Living – Created in 2012, this program supports the ability of people with disabilities and elderly people to remain within their communities, rather than becoming institutionalized. This program initially combined the Administration on Aging, Department on Disability, and Administration on Developmental Disabilities, but has since added on multiple additional programs, all of which fit within the theme of independence and community living.

Adjusted Gross Income – Income calculation used by the IRS, which removes certain credits from your gross income before calculating the taxes you owe.

ADL – Activities of Daily Living – The things people do on a daily basis as part of living life. ADLs include ambulating (ability to move), grooming (personal hygiene), toileting, dressing, and eating. These are activities abled people tend to take for granted. One of the more complicated and emotionally exhausting forms from Social Security's disability application is primarily focused on the applicant's ADL and related social activities.

Affordable Housing – Both title and descriptor, many states and counties are not creative when titling the program to provide assistance to low-income individuals in need of housing assistance. Usually, you will find a variety of resources under this title.

American Rescue Plan, the – Covid-19 stimulus package designed to help the American population and economy recover from the economic damage caused by Covid-19.

Apparent disability – A disability obvious to the casual viewer. Often referred to as visible disability, which often includes blindness (indicated by usage of white cane and/or eye difference), limb difference or absence, Down Syndrome, developmental damage or delay, and anything else that can be immediately recognized by the naked eye, whether it be the condition itself or the use of a disability aid.

ATRC – Accessible Transportation Resource Center – Created in 2022 as part of the ACL. This program focuses on transportation accessibility, not only for disabled and elderly people, but for both historically underserved populations and the general population. This includes not only the transportation system itself, but information about the system and ways to access that information.

Autoimmune Pernicious Anemia – A specific form of pernicious anemia (low B-12) where the immune system attacks the intrinsic factor in the stomach and intestinal lining, preventing the digestive system from moving vitamin B-12 into the bloodstream.

Bankruptcy – Legal process of declaring oneself financially insolvent in order to have debts discharged. There are multiple forms of bankruptcy, and they generally require legal representation and there are expenses involved in the process. This process does not discharge all forms of debt.

Biopsychosocial model – Looking at an interaction or process through the lens of understanding the biological, psychological, and social pressures behind it.

Blue Book – Social Security's guide for medical professionals on the criteria for determining patient disability, focusing on singular systems within the body (such as the skeletal or nervous system).

Break-even Point – With SSI benefits, your break-even point is when you earn enough money that your SSI check would be for $0. To calculate your break-even point, you take your benefit amount, multiply it by 2, then add the $65 earned income allowance and the $20 unearned income allowance. As a formula, that would be (benefit amount) x 2 + $65 + $20. This is a transition point where your Medicaid benefits may be impacted.

Cash surrender value – The amount of money any insurance or investment would be worth if you were to liquidate it now. This is commonly used in any needs-based program. Examples of items with cash surrender value: grave plot purchase, life insurance policy, or savings bonds.

CDFI – Community Development Finance Institution – Private banks created specifically with goals of providing personal lending and business development support in low-income areas. They can receive federal funding from the US Department of Treasury and can also receive funding from other private sources. The goal of these organizations is to provide banking support without bias to communities that commercial banks have traditionally ignored or abused.

Charity Care – Officially often referred to as "financial assistance", this program is found in many hospitals and allows them to reduce hospital bills for low-income patients.

CHIP- Childhood Health Insurance Plan – Medicaid coverage for children under 18. CHIP has similar eligibility standards to Medicaid but is designed specifically for children's needs.

Cisgender – A person whose gender identity aligns with their biological sex. Opposite of Transgender. For example, I was assigned the female identity at birth, and I identify as female. This makes me cisgendered.

Clawbacks – The process of a government program requesting repayment of benefits provided. Over the past 10 years or so, Social Security has been devoting extra effort to reviewing its decisions and payments of SSI, SSDI, and retirement benefits, demanding that beneficiaries repay funds that were paid to them in error or that now appear insufficiently documented.

COBRA – Consolidated Omnibus Budget Reconciliation Act – Federal law passed in 1985 that protects workers' ability to participate in health insurance benefits for a limited additional time after certain life events, such as losing employment, reducing hours, death of a spouse, or divorce.

Community bank – Generally a smaller commercial bank or banking network that serves customers in a relatively small geographic region. These banks are generally more focused on personal relationships and community development and rarely have shareholders to support or consider in their decision-making process.

Community liaison – An individual responsible for building engagement and cultivating relationships between an organization and the community they serve. When hired by a government representative, community liaisons frequently handle questions, complaints, or compliance issues experienced by members of the public, especially when the problem or solution is a government agency.

Glossary » 263

CMS – Centers for Medicare and Medicaid Services – The largest single provider of health insurance in the US, this program manages both Medicare and Medicaid health insurance.

Credit Score – Number that represents your creditworthiness. By far the most commonly used in the US is the FICO score, which ranges from 300-850. The higher your credit score, the more likely you are to get approved for any sort of loan, and the better rate you are likely to get for that loan. Three major credit bureaus in the US (Equifax, Experian, and TransUnion) provide their own FICO score for every person with a credit history.

DAC – Disabled Adult Child – Designation by Social Security Administration for a person who became disabled prior to the age of 22 and is therefore on SSI. The DAC program provides Medicare coverage and SSDI payments to a DAC recipient when their parent retires or dies.

Deductible (insurance) – The amount of money you need to pay before the insurance kicks in. For example, if you have a $50 deductible, you must pay $50 towards the expense before your insurance kicks in the rest of the payment. Most health insurance plans have an annual deductible that you need to spend before your insurance shares the cost. Generally speaking, more expensive insurance plans (ones with higher premiums) have lower deductibles and vice versa.

Deferment – The action or fact of putting something off until a later time. With student loans, this is an official way to put off payments for a limited time period, but debt does accrue while in deferment

DLI – Date Last Insured – The date at which Social Security will no longer consider you eligible for Social Security Disability benefits. SSDI is treated as an insurance policy, so if your payments into the system (taxes from your paycheck or self-employment) stop, the countdown begins for your eligibility for SSDI payments to end.

D. O. – Doctor of Osteopathic Medicine – Meaning they have some differences in their education and some of them may have skills in more manual tasks, like massage, or hands-on work on joints or tissues. They go through the same residency requirements and licensing tests as M.D.s do.

DOL – Department of Labor – Department of the federal government responsible for enforcing labor laws and promoting the general welfare of US wage earners.

Diagnosis – The medical condition/s your doctors agree you have, as documented by the appropriate specialist/s.

DVRS – Division of Vocational Rehabilitation Services – New Jersey's vocational rehabilitation program. They support people with disabilities who are looking to work or return to work. They are generally affiliated with unemployment offices and often are found inside some unemployment offices.

Earned income – Money brought in through your employment or other forms of direct compensation for work products. Compare to unearned income.

EEOC – Equal Employment Opportunities Commission – Government agency responsible for enforcing federal laws regarding discrimination and harassment of employees and job applicants

EPE – Extended Period of Eligibility – For Social Security Disability Insurance coverage. The first 36 months after using up your Trial Work Period with earnings over SGA. During this time, if your income dips below SGA, you notify Social Security, and your checks start up again. After the EPE ends, additional paperwork (referred to as an Expedited Reinstatement) is required

EXR – Expedited Reinstatement – The process of reinstating Social Security Disability benefits following the end of the EPE. For up to 5 years following the end of the EPE, you can notify Social Security of your need for benefits, and payments restart immediately while they investigate your coverage. If you are found ineligible after the fact, they may ask to be reimbursed for these payments.

Fine motor skills (dexterity) – Control over fingers, toes, and other smaller muscle groups. Fine motor issues impact writing, gripping utensils, and other careful coordination of small groups of muscles.

FMLA – Family Medical Leave Act – Federal law protecting employment of people managing a medical or care challenge in their immediate family. It provides protections for up to 12 weeks of unpaid leave to care for self, spouse, child, or parent.

Forbearance – To patiently wait. When referring to loans, it generally means to delay without accruing interest. Student loan forbearances do not accrue interest if your loans are subsidized.

FND – Functional Neurological Disorder – Neurological condition where there is a mis-wiring in the brain, causing neurological symptoms when under certain forms of stress. The symptoms vary widely, and this condition is poorly researched and poorly understood. Previously referred to as conversion disorder and considered a mental illness, FND has now been claimed by the neurological community and the conversion disorder (psychiatric) theory recognized as a partial explanation for some cases of FND.

FPL – Federal Poverty Level – Economic measure used to determine if an individual or family is qualified for certain benefits and programs. The amount is updated annually and based on both household size and geographic location of the household (continental US, Alaska, or Hawaii).

Food desert – A populated area where it's difficult to buy nutritious and affordable food. Often occurs in poor sections of cities and is associated with an increase in diet-related health issues.

Fork (theory) – Forks are the frustrations and challenges you experience that make life harder and increase your risk of emotional meltdown. Like spoons, forks are not an absolute measurement, but more of an acknowledgement of costs. Forks can vary in size, and often removing a fork can make other forks easier to deal with. Examples: "I thought she was my friend, but that pitchfork of intentionally triggering me makes me wonder." "If you want to talk about money, let me hit the bathroom first, I need to pee, and want to get rid of that fork before adding another."

Formulary – List provided by an insurance plan of what medications it covers and what it charges for the medication. Generally, these are divided into tiers with generics and preferred medication on lower tiers (less expensive) and name brands and non-preferred on higher tiers (more expensive)

FY – Fiscal Year – The year based upon the budget. Most calculations (like FPL, federally regulated asset limits, and Social Security's calculations) are for the federal government's fiscal year, which starts October 1 and ends September 30th.

Gaslighting – Pattern of repetitive behavior designed to damage a person's sanity, morality, or sense of self. This can include lying, guilt-tripping, and shaming, but the goal of gaslighting goes beyond the acts themselves to contribute to an abuser's goal of damaging the victim's self-confidence, independence and/or sanity.

Gross Income – Your total amount of income. If you are self-employed, this refers to the total amount of money you earn, and if you have an employer, this generally refers to the amount of money your employer contracted to pay you before taxes and other costs are removed.

Gross motor skills – The interaction of muscles in the limbs and torso, being able to control these muscles and how they interact. Walking, dancing, and other full-body movements, for example, require gross motor coordination.

HHA – Home Health Aide – See PCA, the two terms are frequently used interchangeably, with different states and organizations frequently preferring one over the other.

HMO – Health Maintenance Organization – A type of insurance plan that provides care through a network of providers. HMOs generally have individuals select a Primary Care Physician who refers them to appropriate in-network specialists as needed.

Home and Community Based Care (H&CBC) – This term describes a variety of programs within Medicaid that focus on enabling people who need help and support with one or more aspects of their Activities of Daily Living. Generally, programs are administered on the state or county level. These programs include things like supportive housing, PCA/HHA services (paid in-home care), free transportation, day care programs, and many other unique supports designed to help disabled individuals to stay in their communities rather than being institutionalized. Type and quality of service can vary dramatically between states, as can the wait time for services.

Household – A group of one or more people who reside together and whose pooled income pays living expenses. Example: "We live in a multigenerational household since my mother moved in after she retired and my kids still live here" "My spouse and I are considered two separate households, since we no longer live together." Most needs-based programs use household size and geographic location as considerations for eligibility.

HUD – Department of Housing and Urban Development – Executive department of the US federal government. It is responsible for national policy and programs that address national housing needs, enforces housing regulations, and is intended to improve and develop the nation's communities.

IDR – Income-Driven Repayment (program) – An option for reducing student loan payments. IDR programs use your income as the basis for calculating your repayment, rather than the cost of the loans. Generally, this reduces the amount you pay monthly, and often these programs allow for the discharge of your loan after a certain number of years.

Internalized Ableism – When an individual with a disability views themselves as less human and worthy due to their disability.

IRS – Internal Revenue Service – A division of the US Treasury Department that manages federal taxes.

IRWE – Impairment Related Work Expense – This is a program that reduces your countable earned income based on the financial costs of disability supports that allow you to work. For example, the cost of a Home Health Aide/Personal Care Assistant to help you prepare for work, or a specialized tool or piece of software that allows you to work can be considered IRWEs.

JAN – Job Accommodation Network – A service provided by the DOL's Office of Disability Employment Policy. They provide services to disabled individuals, employers and their representatives, seeking guidance on compliance with ADA regulations, and others who are concerned with successful employment outcomes for individuals with disabilities.

Legislative Liaison – An individual responsible for monitoring and advocating around laws that impact their organization or agency.

LIHEAP – Low Income Heat and Energy Assistance Program – Needs-based federal support program to provide discounted electricity and heating to eligible citizens. Administered on the state level and below.

Living wage – The income amount required to support an individual or family in a particular geographic area. This is in contrast to minimum wage (the lowest amount of money an employer is legally allowed to pay an employee). When the push for a $15/hour minimum wage started, that was an attempt to align minimum wage with the living wage.

Living Will – A legally recognized document that indicates your preferences in medical decisions should you become incapacitated. This may include instructions on whether you wish to be resuscitated should your heart stop beating (often referred to as a DNR), how you would prefer your condition managed, and guidance on your philosophy and perspective on life to help others better understand your desires.

Low-income – Polite way of saying "poor". The precise definition of low-income depends on the specific program or location.

LTD – Long Term Disability – A form of insurance coverage for individuals who become disabled in the long term and are unable to return to work. Industry standard is long term disability coverage kicks in if a person has been unable to work for more than 26 weeks. This insurance can be provided by employers, but is not mandatory, and details will vary.

M.D. – Doctor of Medicine – The medical degree in the United States and some other countries that denotes a medical professional.

Marriage Penalty – Reference to SSI's rules where a single disabled individual can have up to $2,000 in assets, but two SSI recipients who choose to marry (or who "live as married") can only have $3,000 in assets and remain eligible for coverage.

MBSR – Mindfulness-Based Stress Reduction – A practice first described by Jon Kabot-Zimm in 1979 of using mindfulness techniques to help patients manage mental and emotional stresses. Initially this was primarily used to treat and manage pain, but it has since proven useful for many other symptoms/conditions as well. It often combines mindful meditation and yoga to help people better process their life stresses and be less impacted by them than they would otherwise be.

Medicaid – Part of CMS, Medicaid provides healthcare coverage predominantly for low-income individuals. It is managed on a state-by-state basis, with many states now offering expanded coverage for all individuals with income under 133% of the Federal Poverty Level.

Medicaid Threshold Amount – The largest amount of income a disabled individual can have while maintaining eligibility for Medicaid. This value differs between states and is updated annually. It is based on the average Medicaid expenses in that state.

Medical model of disability – The lens or perspective that doctors and other medical professionals often hold when it comes to disability, that there is a specific limitation a person is experiencing, and it is the medical practitioner's responsibility to determine how to get the patient closer to normal functioning. For example, damage to the spine may be solved through wheelchair usage, or psychiatric medication used to stabilize a person whose levels of dopamine or serotonin are consistently off-balance, or nearsightedness can be solved by using glasses with the correct prescription.

Glossary » 269

Medical Power of Attorney – A legal document that empowers another person (referred to as your agent) to make medical decisions for you if you are too ill or otherwise unable to communicate your preferences.

Medical trauma – Physiological or psychological response to a negative or traumatic experience in a medical setting. While it can be caused by the illness, injury, or procedure, it can be caused by the behavior of the medical professionals.

Medicare – Part of CMS, Medicare provides healthcare coverage for recipients of Social Security benefits. This coverage is generally broken down into Parts A (hospital) B (doctor and other medical care not covered by A), D (medication coverage), and C (Medicare Advantage, which allows private insurance companies to handle B and D in one bundle).

Microaggression – A statement, action, or reaction that shows bias (sometimes subconscious) against another individual, generally based on their minority identity. Examples include: misgendering another person (especially if they are trans), a white woman crossing the street at night so she doesn't walk next to a Black man, asking a Native American what country they come from, or assuming an older individual doesn't understand or cannot use technology.

Migraine – Neurological condition, often expressed as a throbbing headache, which generally lasts 4 to 72 hours. It can include nausea, vomiting, and increased sensitivity to light, noise, and/or odors. Some people experience chronic migraines, where these symptoms occur frequently (sometimes continuously), while others experience symptoms of migraine only on occasion.

Moral model of disability – The lens or perspective that disability has a moral value. The significance may be positive or negative. Examples include disabilities being the result of a parent or family member's moral failings, disabilities being a test of an individual's faith (and/or their recovery or survival being due to prayer or passing a moral test), or that prayer will heal a disabled individual.

Myoclonic jerks – Quick, jerking motion in the body outside of conscious control. A hiccup is a form of myoclonic jerk many people experience. Other forms of myoclonus, or myoclonic jerks, are associated with neurological conditions, metabolic conditions, or medication side effects. They can impair ability to eat, speak, or walk, when severe.

Needs-based (programs) – Support based only on financial need. These are social welfare programs that solely require an individual's or household's income to be under some specified amount (usually a percentage of the Federal Poverty Level (FPL)). This would be compared to disability-based or merit-based programs. SNAP and LIHEAP are examples of needs-based programs.

NESE – Net Earned Self-Employment (calculation) – The equation to calculate what Social Security considers your net income while on SSI or SSDI. 0.9235 x (gross income – business expenses) a.k.a. 0.9235 x (net income)

Net income – The amount of money you earn after certain costs have been removed. If you are self-employed, net income usually refers to income after business expenses, and if you have an employer, net income usually refers to the amount on your paycheck, after taxes and related fees have been removed.

Next of Kin – A person's closest living relative or relatives.

Neurodiversity – The perspective that many defined neurological differences (including Autism Spectrum Disorder, ADHD, dyslexia, dyscalculia, and many others) are the result of variations in the human genome, rather than being pathological. In other words, people with these differences are not ill or disordered, but these variations are an essential part of their identity.

Nibling – Gender-neutral term that describes one's sibling's children (equivalent male and female terms are nephew and niece).

Non-apparent disability – A disability is not obvious to the casual viewer. Many disabilities are non-apparent (often referred to as invisible disabilities), including autoimmune disorders, mental illness, fibromyalgia, and many others. This is as opposed to apparent/visible disabilities.

Onset of Disability Date – Social Security's officially recognized month and year in which you became eligible for SSDI or SSI benefits. This determines when Medicare benefits start for SSDI applicants (24 months after this date), whether a child on SSI is eligible for DAC coverage later in life (onset of disability must be before they reached 22 years of age), and how much backpay is owed (backpay starts the month disability started).

Organizational culture – The rules, biases, and norms that exist within any given organization. Organizational culture is usually a combination of stated rules and social interactions.

Pacing – The act of controlling your activities in such a way that you can manage them for a longer period of time, usually a prespecified one. With a disability, pacing often is a long-term process of recognizing your capacity and stopping activities before they trigger a symptom flare or relapse, often switching among physical, mental, and recuperative activities with a long-term goal of preventing flares or relapses.

PASS – Plan to Achieve Self Support – Another tool to manage employment-related expenses. The PASS program allows you to set aside a portion of your disability payment each month to help fund educational opportunities or equipment necessary for you to work. The money set aside through PASS is not considered income, so may leave you eligible for SSI benefits or other financial support while active.

PCA – Personal Care Assistant – An individual paid to support a disabled person in managing their Activities of Daily Living. For example, many full-time wheelchair users may need help with some aspects of toileting, food preparation, eating, personal hygiene, and/or transferring into and out of their chair. PCAs generally do not have medical expertise or professional training. Synonyms include HHA (Home Health Aide) and care attendant.

Personal Injury Protection (PIP) – Known as no-fault car insurance, this is a portion of many car insurance plans that protects the driver and passengers in the event of an accident. It may cover hospital expenses, lost wages, services like childcare, and, if appropriate, funeral expenses.

PHA- Public Housing Authority – A public or governmental organization or agency that develops or operates low-income housing under the United States Housing Act of 1973.

PIA – Principal Insured Amount – A calculation by Social Security, available on your Social Security Statement, which indicates what your monthly payout from Social Security would be if you started collecting benefits now.

Poverty threshold – Used for statistical purposes, a country's poverty threshold is the minimal amount of income viewed as adequate to live in a specific place.

Poverty guidelines – A nation's rules that define poverty in terms of eligibility for specific social welfare programs.

Premium (health insurance) – The amount of money you pay upfront for the service. Generally, your premium is a monthly payment for your health insurance coverage.

Prognosis – The expected outcome of your diagnosis. Prognosis often involves severity of impact, medium-to-long-term expectations, and if the condition is likely to result in death or long-term disability

Progressive condition – Any form of disease or condition that is expected to get worse over time, reducing function or health. Contrast this with a relapsing/remitting condition, where the symptoms sometimes flare up and sometimes plateau or stabilize. With a progressive condition, treatment can slow the progression down, but function or health lost cannot be regained. Examples: Alzheimers, Parkinsons, Osteoarthritis, Muscular Dystrophy

PsyD – Doctor of Psychology – This is a person who has trained to become a clinical psychologist and work with clients or patients to help them manage their mental health

QLE – Qualifying Life Event (insurance) – A qualifying life event is a major change in an insurance recipient's life that qualifies them for a window of time to change or adjust their health insurance plan outside of the open enrollment period. Examples of a qualifying life event include birth, death, or adoption of a covered beneficiary, loss of employment, becoming newly eligible for coverage, or getting a divorce. Generally, the window for a qualifying life event is 45-60 days, depending on the insurance provider.

Red Book – Social Security's guide to employment and working while on SSDI and/or SSI.

Redlining – Historical practice (1930s) of marking particular areas (generally with a red pen/marker) of a community as one where non-white/Black people cannot receive a mortgage or loan towards purchasing property. Used in more recent times to discuss regulations that reinforce the outcomes that redlining encouraged (only allowing non-whites to purchase property in lower-income areas).

Relapsing/Remitting condition – Any form of disease or condition that varies in strength or intensity over time. Often not fully curable, these conditions have variable symptoms that change over time, able to both flare (increase) and decrease at varying points. Neither experience is necessarily permanent, and lost function can often be regained. Contrast this with a progressive condition. Examples: Lupus, Rheumatoid Arthritis.

Representative payee – A person designated responsible for the finances of a disabled person who cannot manage their own. The representative payee receives the beneficiary's monthly check from Social Security with the expectation they will use it to pay for the disabled individual's care and living expenses.

Right to Sue – Referred as full tort (as opposed to limited tort), your ability to sue the other driver in a car accident for pain and suffering (as opposed to just financial costs) is impacted by the plan you choose. Maintaining your right to sue/full tort is an additional expense for many policies. If you do not pay for this right, you can only sue the other driver if the damage is permanent, and only for the financial costs involved.

Same-sex marriage – Referred to as gay marriage (which further marginalizes the Bi+ community), the legal right to marry a person who shares your sex. Same-sex marriage was legally recognized on the federal level in June 2015, after over 40 years of fighting by the LGBTQ community.

SAVE – Saving on a Valuable Education – The newest IDR program, this can allow for total discharge of student loans in as little as 10 years.

Section 8 – Part (Section 8) of the Housing Act of 1973, this allows qualified renters to have a portion of their rental payments be covered by the federal government

Selective (law) enforcement – The practice of only enforcing certain laws under certain circumstances. Often, this is associated with bias, where police or other legal authorities either choose to let the privileged class of people get away with breaking certain laws or only enforcing the laws when people with a disadvantaged identity are seen breaking them. Examples of this include "nuisance" crimes like loitering or jaywalking, private property that is often treated as a common good (unwanted visitors are considered trespassers), or failing to enforce accessibility laws because somebody else should do it.

Self-efficacy – Belief in your own ability, specifically your ability to meet challenges and complete tasks.

Self-employment – Choosing to work independently, rather than having an employer. This can be creating your own business or choosing to do gig work as an independent contractor. When you are self-employed, you are responsible for structuring your business, paying all taxes, and finding your own health insurance. You set your own hours and determine the amount and type of work that you do.

SGA – Substantial Gainful Activity – Social Security's stated amount of earned income above which a person is considered ineligible for disability payments after certain deductions are made. The amount changes annually and is higher for SSDI-eligible people who are legally blind. In 2025, SGA for all SSI and most SSDI recipients is $1,620 and for all blind SSDI recipients is $2,700.

Sliding scale – Pay rate is dependent on income. This process is designed to lower costs for low-income participants. Sometimes the amounts are clearly defined, other times it is more of a pay-as-you-can trust-based system.

SNAP – Supplemental Nutrition Assistance Program – Program run by the US Department of Agriculture to provide funds specifically for the purchase of food to low-income households, including elderly and disabled individuals. Needs-based program available throughout the US, While the program is national, it is administered at the state or tribal level, sometimes by individual counties or cities.

SOAR – SSI/SSDI Outreach, Access, and Recovery – Run by the Substance Abuse and Mental Health Services Administration, this educational model trains caseworkers to help individuals with mental illness or substance use disorders, especially those who are homeless or at risk of homelessness, to apply for SSI and/or SSDI. They provide information resources on applying for these programs.

Social model of disability – The perspective or belief that disability is a social construct (an identity created by society) and so it is society's responsibility to make spaces accessible to people with disabilities.

Social Enterprise – Business with social objectives that serve as its primary purpose. Many focus on one or more at-risk communities and frequently hire within those communities or otherwise ensure those communities benefit directly from their work. Social enterprises are businesses which focus on being financially sustainable, but balance that with their social objective. Examples of social enterprises include Warby Parker (provides a free pair of glasses to a person in need for every pair sold) and Bitty & Beau's Coffee (coffee shop that employs people with intellectual and developmental disabilities with the goal of ensuring those employees have meaningful employment and a sense of belonging while educating and inspiring customers).

Social Signature – Each person's number of close friendships they can naturally maintain, with other relationships being considered social acquaintances. Social signatures are considered stable, but I would argue many disabilities decrease many things viewed as constants in the study, indicating that part of the loneliness people with disabilities experience is partially due to no longer being able to maintain their social signature.

Spoon (theory) – Spoons are units of emotional and physical energy required to get things done. Used within disability communities as a shorthand when discussing tasks and plans. Examples: "I went for a walk yesterday, but today I didn't have the spoons." or "I'm watching my spoons this week because I want to go to the conference on Friday!"

SSA – Social Security Administration – Government agency that handles retirement and disability financial programs, including SSI, SSDI, and Social Security Retirement Benefits.

SSI – Supplemental Security Income – The other "disability" program administered by the Social Security Administration. This program is specifically for poor disabled and elderly people who do not have the work history to be eligible for SSDI.

SSDI – Social Security Disability Insurance – Often referred to as "disability", this program provides Social Security benefits to people unable to perform substantial gainful activity (SGA) due to disability and too young to be eligible for retirement benefits.

Stigma – Mark of disgrace, associated with a particular circumstance, quality, or person.

Structural Ableism – Physical and social structures that prevent the full participation of disabled people in society. Parallel to structural racism and sexism, structural ableism can be seen throughout society but is rarely considered by abled people. Examples include places only accessible by stairs, alarm systems only accessible through one sense, employment applications that are not fully accessible, and the many biases that equate disability with inability to work.

Structural Racism – Social structures (and physical barriers) that prevent full participation of non-whites (especially Black people) in society. Historical examples include slavery, segregation, and redlining, and modern examples include police bias against Black people, medical professionals assuming Black people have higher pain tolerance than white people, and the tendency of employers to reject job applications with "black-sounding" names when compared to identical applications from "white-sounding" names.

Supported Decision Making – A set of legal protections for people with disabilities who cannot completely direct their own care or manage their money. Every state has slightly different laws around Supported Decision Making, but this process protects and/or empowers individuals with disabilities who may need some form of guardianship put in place as adults.

Supportive housing – Programs that combine affordable housing with the appropriate coordinated support services, which allows residents (often people with disabilities) to have stable, affordable housing and better manage their conditions. Generally, these programs are for people who cannot live independently.

TANF – Temporary Assistance for Needy Families – Federal program administered on the state level to provide financial support for low-income families. The program now cannot extend beyond 5 years of support.

Temporary Disability Coverage – Insurance that covers a disabling event anticipated to take a relatively short period of time to recover from. While a few states provide temporary disability coverage, it is usually the employer's responsibility and is usually considered optional rather than being legally required. Industry standard definition of temporary disability is 26 weeks or fewer, but details will vary.

Threshold amount – The maximum amount of income permitted before eligibility for a program ends.

Ticket to Work – Social Security program designed to help people collecting SSI or SSDI benefits train for and/or find appropriate work opportunities.

Total and Permanent Disability Discharge – Program that allows an individual who has been disabled for 5 years or longer or is anticipated to have a disability that prevents them from earning substantial income for the rest of their life to have their entire student loan forgiven.

Toxic positivity – The belief that no matter how difficult a situation is, people must maintain a positive mindset.

Transgender – Person whose gender identity does not align with their biological sex. Opposite of cisgender. For example, Elliot Page was assigned the female identity as birth, and initially named Ellen, but he has come out as transgender.

Trauma – Deeply distressing or disturbing experience, or physical injury.

Treatment plan – Ideally created through collaboration, a treatment plan lays out what the doctor and patient agree are the necessary steps for the understanding and management of the patient's condition/s. Some doctors will create a treatment plan without patient input. Examples: "My neurologist and I agreed on my treatment plan: I'm going to try this new CGRP inhibitor for the next month and track my headaches to see how much it helps. I also have to pick up sunglasses to protect my eyes on the days I'm light-sensitive." "My doctor needs me to get an MRI and a DEXA scan to complete their diagnosis, and I'm scheduled to see them the following week to create the next steps of my treatment plan."

TWL – Trial Work Level – A specified amount of income that increases annually. If a person on SSDI earns under this amount of income, they can continue at that pay rate without risk to their benefits. Once they earn that amount or over in the course of a month, they use up one month of their Trial Work Period. The TWL for 2025 is $1,160.

TWP – Trial Work Period – A period of 9 months during which a person on SSDI can earn any amount of money without losing their Social Security benefits. Any month with income over the TWL (Trial Work Level) counts as one month of the Trial Work Period. Trial Work months do not need to be consecutive and are accumulated as long as there are 5 years or less between Trial Work months. Once the TWP is completed, the EPE (Extended Period of Eligibility) countdown begins.

Unearned income – Income that is not the direct result of work or work products. This can include Social Security payments, dividends from investments,

Universal Design – Design concept focused on making products or spaces accessible and usable by everybody, regardless of age, ability, or other factors.

Urinary urgency – Medical symptom set where the patient frequently experiences the need to pee, even when they have just done so, or could not have filled their bladder so quickly.

USDA – United States Department of Agriculture – An executive department of the United States of America, which provides leadership on food, agriculture, rural areas, nutrition, and related issues.

Vocational Rehabilitation – Funded by the Department of Education, these programs exist in every state, territory, and many Indian Nations. The goal of this program is to help people with disabilities to prepare for, obtain, and maintain paid employment.

WIC – Women, Infants, and Children – Needs-based program to provide affordable food to mothers and their (young) children

Work – Effort put forth to achieve a necessary goal. While it is casually used to equate to employment, unpaid work is common and essential for society to function. Examples include household maintenance (like laundry, food preparation, balancing finances, and washing dishes), childcare, maintaining your household's health, eldercare, proving eligibility for appropriate support programs, and filing taxes.

Work culture – The combination of attitudes, beliefs and behaviors that make up a work environment. Examples include formality (or informality) of dress, preferred modes of communication, attitudes about work/life balance, and (the awareness of) bias in the work environment. Every office has a work culture, the question is how comfortable you are in your workplace and how accepting it is of your disability (and other identities).

Workability (NJ) – New Jersey program to support people with disabilities who wish to work. It guarantees Medicaid benefits to participants at any income level if they are determined disabled. Those above a certain income level will pay a premium for these benefits. Effectively, this program allows NJ residents with disabilities to not need to fear becoming uninsured due to earned income.

Workers' Compensation - Employers provide workers' compensation, a form of disability insurance, to assist employees injured on the job. Legally required in all states but Texas.

www.ingramcontent.com/pod-product-compliance
Lightning Source LLC
Chambersburg PA
CBHW052028030426
42337CB00027B/4908